THE MYSTERY Of Mind

DR K M DRUVA KUMAR,
M.B.B.S, DABPsych(USA)

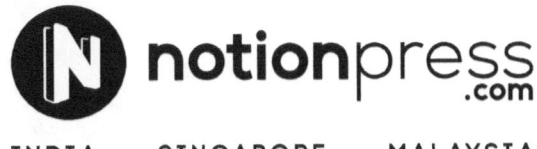

INDIA • SINGAPORE • MALAYSIA

Notion Press

No.8, 3rd Cross Street
CIT Colony, Mylapore
Chennai, Tamil Nadu – 600004

First Published by Notion Press 2021
Copyright © Dr K M Druva Kumar, M.B.B.S, DABPsych(USA) 2021
All Rights Reserved.

ISBN 978-1-63781-487-1

This book has been published with all efforts taken to make the material error-free after the consent of the author. However, the author and the publisher do not assume and hereby disclaim any liability to any party for any loss, damage, or disruption caused by errors or omissions, whether such errors or omissions result from negligence, accident, or any other cause.

While every effort has been made to avoid any mistake or omission, this publication is being sold on the condition and understanding that neither the author nor the publishers or printers would be liable in any manner to any person by reason of any mistake or omission in this publication or for any action taken or omitted to be taken or advice rendered or accepted on the basis of this work. For any defect in printing or binding the publishers will be liable only to replace the defective copy by another copy of this work then available.

Contents

Foreword   5

Foreword   7

Preface   15

1. The Mysterious Mind   19
2. Flower Phobia   28
3. Fear of Death   33
4. Guilt   40
5. Social Media Addiction   44
6. Examination Fear   48
7. Worrying Syndrome   51
8. Hypochondriasis   57
9. Sun Allergy   64
10. Inferiority Complex   71
11. Poor Concentration   79
12. Narrow Mindedness   83
13. Being Poisoned   89
14. Bad Omen   94

Contents

15. Pinching Disease	103
16. Mind Reading	107
17. Breathlessness and Palpitation	110
18. Body Odour	116
19. Grief Reaction	125
20. Gambling	132
21. Selfishness	139
22. Cramps	144
23. Allergy	152
24. Fear of Devil	159
25. Obsessive Compulsive Disorder	165
26. Attacks of Pulling Sensation	172
27. Living In The Past	179
28. Greed	184
29. Paralysis	190
30. Paranoid Delusion	197
31. Uncontrolled Neck Movements	201
32. Transgender	207
33. Bipolar Disorder	212
34. Do You Have A Mental Illness?	215
About the Author	*221*

Foreword

Dr.V.A.P.Ghorpade,
B.Sc., M.B., B.S., D.P.M., M.D.
Consultant Psychiatrist,
Rtd Prof & HOD of Psychiatry from
M.S.R.Medical College, Banglaore & AIMS, Bellur cross, Mandya Dt.

With great pleasure and enthusiasm, I agreed to the author's request to write a foreword for his book entitled "The Mysteries of Mind" and started going through the book. Cover page is the most creative art, giving a hint to the reader, that journey into mind (of the author as well many of his patients) is going to be an interesting adventure.

"Searching the sky with satellites, one does not find God, and scanning the brain tissue under the microscope one does not find the mind" thus Dr.Sarvapalli Radhakrishnan, former president of India and great teacher and philosopher, expressed. Mind cannot be seen but through indirect means such as subjective description by psychiatric patients, experiencing the working of the mind by all individuals, and other methods, one can understand the "Mind". Hence the title of the book is aptly titled as "The Mysteries of Mind".

Whole book is organized in a systematic way so that first chapter deals with the structure and function of mind as understood by psychoanalysts and psychotherapists. Subsequent chapters deal with the various kinds of Psychiatric patients which all psychiatrists deal with it very frequently. In the eyes of a common man these kinds of cases will be an enigma. In Hindu spiritual literature, six causes are recognized as the root cause of human misery, and they are Kama,

Krodha, Lobha, Madha, Mathsaraya and Moha. Similarly, all cases which are narrated in this book, are related to one or more than one factors mentioned above. The task of a psychiatrist is to find out the root cause of these anomalies as patients present themselves or as brought by their relatives with problems related to either body, mind or both. Psychiatrist patiently listens to the narration, non-judgmentally chronologically analyzes the events and try to create a network. Missing links are probed with an artful questioning and fill up the gaps, so that, patient is made to become aware of the TRUTH. In other words, whole psychiatric consultation and management is nothing but truth finding. Psychiatrist is peace giver to the one who does not have peace of mind. Then why stigma of psychiatric illness and consultation with a psychiatrist is so strong in our society? All points to prevalence of a dark cloud of ignorance, which can be cleared only with knowledge and Education, which has been covered in detail in the last chapter of this book. Thus, this journey ended with a sign of happiness and giving rise to a wish that this book can help both society and other junior doctors and psychiatrists to refine their skills so that, Peace in the mind of people prevails, and society health will be optimum. I hope my experiences while reading this book will also be echoed in the mind of other readers

(Dr.V.A.P.Ghorpade)
ghorpade.vap@gmail.com

Foreword

Mind: We can't see and we can't touch it.

Mind directs our thinking, emotions, actions and reactions – total behaviors.

Mind motivates us to take care of our basic needs like hunger, thirst, sleep, sex, protection. Mind also creates and takes care of our desires, ambitions, aspirations and goals.

Mind understands the experiences of our five senses, learns and stores information for later use. It is also responsible for our knowledge ,attitudes and decisions.

Mind has creativity, safeguards or destroys. Mind makes and breaks friendship and relationships.

Mind makes us to kill or commit suicide!

Mind makes man a God or a monster!!

Upanishad

ಮನ ಏವ ಮನುಷಾಯ ಣಾಂ ಕಾರಣಂ ಬಂಧ ಮೋಕಷ ಯೋಃ!

ಬಂಧಾಯ ವಿಷಯಾಸಕತಂ ಮುಕಾತಂ ನಿವಿಷಯಂ ಸಮೃತಮ್!!

Mind makes man attached to passions and relationships, mind can make man detached from desires, passions and thrive for liberation (mukthi/moksha)

Extensive research has been done by Indian thinkers about Mind

Vedic period (10000 – 5000 B.C)

Mind is the functional part of Athma (Soul). Athma is the supreme inner energy of man. Pure mind was believed to lead towards positive health.

"RIGVEDA" describes 3 types of mind or personality – Satvik, Rajasik and Thamasik.

Satvik Mind is full of love, kindness, peace. It makes the person to lead simple and harmonious life. No selfishness. He/she works for the welfare of others and society.

Rajasik mind is full of desires, ambitions. Drives man to go behind money, power and luxuries. He/she dictates others and wants them to obey and serve them.

Thamasik mind is full of ignorance, laziness, entertains superstitious beliefs, acts foolishly, no goals/aspirations.

"YAJURVEDA" describes mind as "Inner light of knowledge", and has 2 stages – Jagrutha and Swapna (fully awake & dreamy state)

"ATHARVANA VEDA" describes sick mind – unmaada (madness)- abnormal thinking, emotions, behaviors and illusion. It prescribes medicines, prayers, chanting hymns, exorcism (driving away evil forces), music, dance as treatment.

UPANISHAD describes 4 stages of mind – Jagrutha, Swapna, Sushuptha and Samadhi.

    9 mental powers (shakthi)

1. Volition   -   (Ichcha shakthi)
2. Action   -   (Kriya shakthi)
3. Knowledge   -   (Jnana shakthi)
4. Sensation   -   (vedana)

5. Memory   -   (Jnapaka)
6. Emotions   -   (Bhava)
7. Decision   -   (Manisha)
8. Determination -   (Sankalpa)
9. Dharana   -   (concentration)

VEDANTHA makes athma as supreme which has 3 wings :-

1. Body with sensory and working organs (Jnanendriya's – karmendriya's)
2. Mind with emotions and passions
3. Intelligence (Buddhi) with thoughts either realistic and/or worldly.

AYURVEDA (Charaka and Sushrutha) (1500 to 1400 BC)

It declares – "Prasanna kaya (body), mana (mind), indriya (sensory organs) and Athma lead to total health".

Kama (desires), krodha (anger), lobha (collecting wealth), moha (passion/excess attachment), mada (excess pride), maathsarya (jealousy), shoka (grief), chinthe (worries), chittodreka (excitement) are causes of mental ill health.

To improve mental health, Ayurveda suggests :-

i. Celibacy (Brahmacharya – control of sexual needs)
ii. Knowledge (Jnana)
iii. Donation (Daana)
iv. Be happy with what you get
v. Remain peaceful (Shaanthi)
vi. Friendship

Foreword

"PATANJALI's ASHTANGA YOGA" helps in "Chitta Vritthi Nirodha" -Control your thoughts, desires, fantasy, memories, experience by :-

a) Yama – Niyama

b) Shoucha – swadhyaya – eswari pranidana

c) Asana

d) Pranayama

e) Prathyahara

f) Dharana

g) Dhyana

h) Samadhi

MODERN UNDERSTANDING OF MIND

Mind doesn't exist at the time of birth. A newborn child cannot understand what it sees or hears. It can't think, it can't express emotions. Except for reflex actions for pain it can't show any meaningful responses. Mind develops over a period of 20 years, based on several factors like:-

i. Genetic factors.

ii. Nutrition

iii. Parenting :- Love and discipline

iv. Family – environment

v. People in and around

vi. School – classmates – teachers.

vii. Media and models

viii. Socio-cultural factors

ix. Positive and negative life events and experiences

x.   Reward and punishment

xi. Health and ill health

xii. Norms, ethics, values etc....

One may have strong and efficient mind; another may have weak and insufficient mind.

Thus, each person develops a mental-set and personality which is unique to oneself. Children of same parents and family act and react differently to both positive and negative life events.

By nature, mind is usually unstable, and its reactions can be unpredictable. Its equilibrium gets disturbed with trivial stimuli or stress but may take long time to come back to normal state. Thoughts, emotions and behavior may become negative causing distress to the individual or to others. One needs counselling and guidance, but in our country, there are very limited Psychiatrists, Psychologists (less than 6000 for a country with population of more than 130 crores)

Mental disorders are of various shades and types, some are very minor, and some are very serious. According to International Classification Diseases (ICD) there are more than 300 different mental disorders. Severe mental disorders arise out of chemical changes in the brain. Minor mental disorders are the result of internal stress or external stress. Stress may be in the area of self-esteem, lack of coping skills, family and interpersonal relationships, finance, job or conflicts with ethical, legal and social norms. Severe mental disorders require medicines whereas minor mental disorders may require psychotherapy or counselling and good relaxation.

In our country, people find it difficult to accept mental disorders and don't approach professionals for treatment. They feel comfortable seeking help and guidance from religious, spiritual, traditional healers because they attribute all mental aberrations to supernatural forces, planetary movements, ghosts, black magic or sorcery or vaasthu.

Because of social stigma attached to mental ailments equating them to "madness or insanity', they somatize their psychological distress into bodily symptoms. They start complaining about one or many bodily symptoms like pain, weakness, fatigue, numbness, indigestion, constipation, tremors and take up a sick role. They get sympathy from family members and get work concessions or at least attention from hostile spouse or in laws. They go to any medical person for investigation and treatment. Studies have revealed prevalence of somatization as 5% in general population and 30 to 40% people who seek medical help either in govt hospitals/private clinics or hospitals. They refuse to accept the psychogenicity of their symptoms.

Somatization is a process in which an inappropriate focus is on physical symptoms and psycho-social problems are denied. As there are secondary gains in terms of reduced work responsibilities and caring responses by the family members, they remain believing that they are physically ill! This belief is enforced and encouraged by general doctors and investigatory labs for their gains!

It becomes an uphill task for Psychiatrists to convince these patients to accept Psychiatric treatment. Drop out rate is very high.

As people are made to believe in **"Karma Theory"**, they have a fixed idea that mental disorders are due to past bad deeds of previous life and expect religious rituals, surrendering themselves to God of their choice for getting relief from the disorder! They request religious leaders to meditate!

The pathway study done in India revealed that Psychiatrist is the 10th or 11th agency to be approached for treatment. The first five to six agencies are temples, dargah's, churches', astrologers, faith healers. Certain popular shrines attract thousands of mentally ill for help even today!

In 1970's and 80's, people did not want me to write my name or put NIMHANS seal on the envelope but sought my suggestion or guidance for their mental ailments. They thought a letter from NIMHANS carry stigma and they get looked down by neighbors. I wrote more than 30,000 letters doing postal counselling.

Dr.K.M.Dhruvakumar is senior to me, I met him in Indian Psychiatric Society's meet which took place in Nandi Hills. Coming to know that he practices Psychodynamic Psychotherapy my respect towards him doubled. I used to read his articles in Kasthuri monthly digest and appreciated his writings. I found him very friendly.

In spite of age difference and seniority, Dr.KMD and his better half became good friends of my wife & myself. He instituted an award for Psychotherapy done by P.G.students in his name. He used to take active part in I.P.S meets. He became President for one term.

Many patients treated by him used to speak highly about him. Les or no medicine, but only talking treatment. Some were unhappy when there was delay in improvement. This happens to all Psychiatrists in our country, as people expect instantaneous miracle cure!

He has sustained his interest in doing Psychotherapy when majority of Psychiatrist have given up, restricting themselves to pharmacotherapy which is easy and less time consuming. I call them as "prescribing machines"!.

He rang me a couple of days ago and wanted me to write a foreword for his book "The Mystery of Mind", which he wrote using COVID-19 time!. He has given a detailed account of 31 case stories which makes a very interesting reading. Like a detective, he has succeeded in revealing hidden or forgotten stress factors causing the ailments. He has unearthed the secrets of mind of clients.

Foreword

One may wonder and exclaim "is it so"? (ಹೇಗೂ ಉಂಟೆ?) and keep one's finger on the nose!

At the end of the book he gives tips to the readers regarding symptoms of mental disorders. His language, style of presentation, narration are simple and can be easily understood by common man. One may even complete the reading at one stretch!

I thank him for this good work and expect many more such books both in English and Kannada as he is retired from clinical work and has free time to do so.

I wish that the book finds a place in every house, not only in Karnataka but every part of India.

Let everybody enjoy good health and "Ananda"

Dr. C.R.Chandrashekar
Retd Professor
Deputy Medical Superintendent, Dept of Psychiatry,
NIMHANS, Bengaluru. 560 079
Founder Trustee
SAMADHANA Centre for Counselling and Guidance
Bengaluru – 560 076

Preface

My interest in emotional problems began while I was interning at KR hospital about 55 years ago. Just like anybody new in the profession my enthusiasm and inquisitiveness were high. My teachers were excellent. Despite the best treatment some patients didn't have adequate relief from their symptoms. When those patients stopped me and talked to me about their personal problems there was a relief in their symptoms. For the first time I realized the importance of the role of mind in physical ailments. I decided to pursue my further training in psychiatry.

I completed my residency and fellowships in Wayne state university in USA. After passing American board of psychiatry examination I became a full-fledged psychiatrist. I was on faculty at Wayne state university. I was the first Indian to be selected to Michigan psychoanalytic institute. I was also on the hospital staff of Hurley Hospital in Flint, Michigan. I was also Director of Drug Abuse Unit, Detroit, Michigan. I always longed to return to India. My attachment to my country was very intense.

The very first thing I noticed in India was an immense stigma and ignorance about emotional problems. The trend was to label all emotional problems as madness. People feared emotionally ill people. The media were projecting all emotionally ill people as crazy. The movies displayed emotionally ill people as acting strange in a peculiar manner. In practice I had a personal experience of the enormity of the stigma. I had many incidences to quote, but I will quote only one such example. Once a couple visited me. I recognized them. I had treated their daughter. They thanked me once again saying their daughter completed studies (She wanted to discontinue her studies before coming to me). Her marriage was fixed, and they gave me an invitation. I thanked them. While they were about to leave, they said sheepishly "Doctor don't mistake us, this is invitation for your information only. If you come people start wondering why you came and what is the relationship between you and us. If they come to know that you are a psychiatrist, they may even label our daughter as insane. The marriage may even break up". I told them that I understood the situation and wouldn't attend.

Being aware of the enormity of the stigma I felt that I should contribute towards the society to thwart the ignorance. I began writing articles on mental illness. I thought the best way to reach people was to present actual cases taking adequate precaution to safeguard their identities. I published many articles in "Kasthuri", a kannada magazine. It was well received by people. I compiled all those articles and published as a book by name "Manoviplava"in1997. Since then I had lot more experience and decided to add a greater number of cases and bring out a second edition to it. I also wanted to bring it out in English for the sake of non-Kannadigas.

I also got associated with Indian Psychiatric society, Karnataka branch. I was active and a member, Executive committee member, Treasurer and finally president. My association with other psychiatrists was very memorable. Even though I was never a student or a staff of Nimhans, I had the full support of each one of them. I had several awards from Indian psychiatric society, Karnataka. The most important was Eminent Psychiatrist award in 1997-98. The same year I was given the honor of being the Chairman for the annual conference of the society. I was a recipient of Dr LGP Achar, Dr SS Jayaram and Senior psychiatrist awards. I was a recipient of

Community leaders award in USA. I was also recipient of Two Rotary Awards.

My patients were my source of information. It was a very satisfying experience. I have learnt a lot by treating them. What can be more satisfying? I must express sincere thanks to them. I also would like to thank my wife, Gayathri and children for their support.I would like to thank Dr C R Chandrashekhar and Dr V A P Ghorpade for the forewords.

In this book there are 35 chapters with 31 actual case summaries with description of treatment and outcome. This is to alleviate ignorance and stigma on mental ailments in general public. There are chapters on Mind's structure and functions, Examination fear, Etc. **The confidentiality of the patient is protected.** The last chapter helps the reader to self- assess and decide if a person needs Psychiatric intervention.

This book may be helpful to general public, medical students, general practitioners, Trainees in psychiatry and psychology, etc.

The adage "mental illness is not curable" is a myth. It is curable.

Dr K M Druva Kumar

The Mysterious Mind

Ramu is my childhood friend. He says that he doesn't understand his own mind. When we are together, he is deeply engrossed in some thoughts, which he doesn't want but seem to be intruding his mind. He asks why these unwanted thoughts keep intruding his mind. Raja Rao is my club friend. He says that his mind is splintered, and he has no control over his mind. Venkatappa is my patient. He says he has no peace of mind and can't sleep properly. Sharadamma has many physical symptoms for three years. She has seen many specialists, and all have declared that she had no physical illness. Her question is if she has no physical illness then why she has physical symptoms. She blames doctors for not able to cure her. She was fed up of life. People like Ramu, Raja Rao, Venkatappa and Sharadamma are in plenty. What is the problem of all these people? Is it physical, psychological or both? Hopefully my future chapters of case treatment narration may throw some light to the readers.

Our body is one and has different parts. If one part of the body fails to function, it is compensated to a certain extent by another part. This is called as compensation. If a person is affected with polio of right leg, the left leg bears additional stress and those muscles will become strong to bear additional stress. There is a limit for compensation also. If it exceeds the limit, it may cause problems. Just like our body our mind also has different parts and the principle of compensation applies here also. Mind cannot be seen and hence its parts also. If we understand our thoughts and actions, we can understand our minds.

Sigmund Freud was the first person to make mind and its problems understandable. He was from Austria. He was a neurologist. In his practice he experienced that some patients wouldn't get better despite the best treatment. He realized that there was more to just the body i.e. mind. He underwent training with Chacot and Liebolt to learn more about the functioning of the mind. Then he began using hypnosis on those patients who were not improving. In the practice of hypnosis Freud learnt more on the existence of unconscious mind. The effect of hypnosis treatment was excellent but soon Freud realized that hypnosis was curing his patients only temporarily.

The effect of hypnosis was short lived. The effect was wearing off in a short period. He discontinued the practice of hypnosis. He began instructing his patients to talk anything and everything that came to their minds, without reservation and in a conscious state. He later labeled it as Free association. The experience in hypnosis and free association made Freud realize that mind also has different parts. He called them unconscious, Conscious and pre conscious. He called this as topographical theory. We are aware of the conscious mind. The unconscious mind is not usually available to our awareness. The preconscious mind is not available for awareness usually, but available easily for conscious mind within a few moments. In any decision that we take all the three parts of mind will be interacting. Often people ask for the evidence for the existence of unconscious mind. Sometimes we tell ourselves not to do a thing and end up doing that only. At the end we wondered how we could do it and say there was some force beyond our control. This is exactly the unconscious mind.

Freud also propagated another theory called structural theory. He said that mind has three different parts viz: - ID, Ego and Superego. He called this as structural theory. With the promulgation of these two theories Freud made mind understandable.

Topographical theory

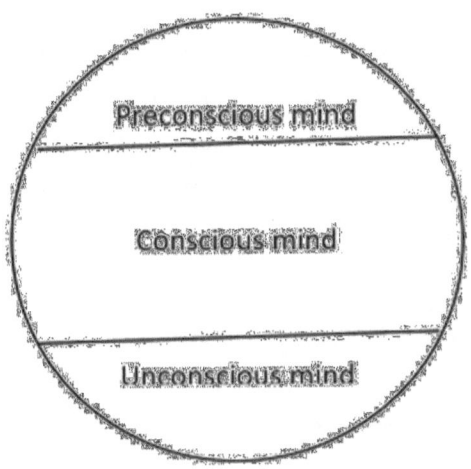

Structural theory

ID is full of natural instincts and it is primitive. It has no controls, no morals, no order and no sense of right and wrong; opposites can exist at the same time and has no sense of time. Superego is the moral aspect of the mind. It is inculcated from parents, other elders, teachers, etc. Ego is the adult part. It mediates between Id and Superego. Ego takes the final decision.

With the promulgation of these two theories the birth of psychoanalysis took place. Psyche means mind and analysis means understanding of the mind. This treatment involved 5 sessions a week and lasted for 5 to 10 years and even more also. It was an exhaustive treatment; the entire unconscious mind of the patient was explored. The critics of psychoanalysis felt that this lengthy treatment was not suitable in this fast world. They began to think what the necessity was to explore the entire unconscious mind. The result was emergence of psychodynamic psychotherapy. It is a shorter therapy of 8 to 10 sessions. It is a symptom-oriented therapy. The unconscious mind's exploration is limited to understand the root cause of the symptom and give relief to the patient. This can be best understood if I give you an analogy. If you have trouble of the brakes in your car the mechanic can just fix the breaks and send you (this is Psychodynamic psychotherapy). The other way is for the mechanic to check each part of the car (this is psychoanalysis). In the process of exhaustive checking something else may go wrong. In the same way analyzing the entire mind may evoke disturbance in another part of the mind.

The post Freudian era brought further changes. Shorter psychotherapy emerged. They are called as psychotherapies. These are symptom-oriented therapies. One form of psychotherapy is psychodynamic psychotherapy. Here the root cause of the symptom is explored and brought into the conscious mind of the patient. Psychodynamic psychotherapy is used mostly by me in my practice. Generally, we do not stick to one method in our clinical practice and we may use multiple modes to give relief to the patient.

Eric Berne tried to make the mind easy to understand. He said that we have three parts in mind viz: - child, Parents and Adult. It is somewhat like Freud's structural theory. This may represent ID superego and ego respectively of Freud. He coined the term Transactional analysis. The interaction between two people is a transaction and analysis of transactions will lead to better coping mechanism of the ego.

Transaction analysis of Eric Berne   Structural theory of Freud

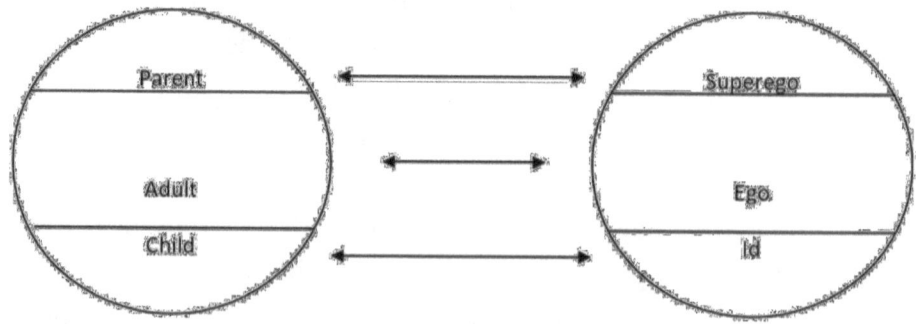

At birth child has only ID instincts. As he grows, he is exposed to the moral values of the parents. Supposing a child tares a paper, immediately the parents say "no". The child incorporates parental values. Still at a later age child may say it is wrong to tare the paper even if it is for a good reason. He, himself doesn't know what is right or wrong, he just inculcates what the parents have taught blindly. He has not yet developed discretionary mind of his own. He is more exposed to "No" than "Yes" as a child; this is the reason why a child learns to say "no" before he learns to say "yes". This is the beginning of superego. Gradually child develops his own mind to become an adult. In the process he asks questions why it is wrong or right. This is an intermediary process towards adulthood. Further it will lead to develop his own individuality to become an adult. As an adult he develops his own independent mind and values.

At this stage in a child there is only ID and Superego. The Ego is yet to develop. If a child (ID) wants to do something the Superego may say "no" for that. The child begins to think why it is right or wrong. This is the beginning of the development of Ego. As the child grows further into an adult, he will have his own definite value systems. We call this as individuality. He develops unique ideas and values. In a mature individual Id, Superego and Ego interact together and arrive at a harmonious decision.

Our conscious thoughts are an interaction of all the three parts of our mind. If someone sees some delectable item in a shop, Id (child) part will say go and grab it. The Superego (Parent) will say not to do it. Then Ego (adult) will recognize the demands of both and mediate to arrive at a more acceptable solution. Ego may say buy it and be happy. Let us say Ego has not developed properly in a person, and then he may grab it and get into trouble and feel bad for doing it (Superego). In a mature individual a normal conflict like this is well solved by a mature Ego in a mature way. If Ego development is not mature the conflict is not solved. He may act in one way or other and gets into trouble. If the conflict persists it will lead to anxiety and may result in further psychological problems.

The ID is full of psychic energy. Which Freud called as Libido. It is not unlimited. It is generated in an ongoing basis. This energy is responsible for our achievements. When the energy is utilized in a constructive way it is called as sublimation. If this energy is wasted in Psychological problems, that much energy availability for sublimation is less. That person achieves less in life. If the psychological conflict is not solved, it will generate anxiety. This may lead to all types of mental illness. Everybody has both good and bad thoughts. Some people try to force these thoughts out of consciousness, but they are going to be back after some time. Mind should be free to think of anything, even bad thoughts. Our controls should be on action.

Human being is a very intelligent person. Sometimes the reason for a given act may not be the real one. Let us say someone says he hates a person, because of his caste. If we explore deep we will know that he has some other friends from the same caste. The real reason for his hatredness for that person is not caste, but something else in his unconscious mind.

Every action is a result of interaction of conscious and unconscious minds. Our reactions are sometimes reflective of our unconscious mind. If two people are asked for their reaction, when shown a glass half filled with water, one may say it is half full and another may say it is half empty, both are correct technically. First one is an optimist and second one is a pessimist.

Our mind is influencing our vision, hearing, etc also. A mother wakes up for the shrill voice of her baby and not for other louder sounds at work in the factory. We call this selective hearing. This is achieved through Reticular activating system of our central nervous system. Our mind commands this tract to let in only what it desires (it may be conscious or unconscious command). This is the mystery of mind.

There is a normal and harmoniously functioning (homeostasis) mind and on the other hand disturbed functioning of the mind in mental illness. There is an intermediary phase to it also. Whenever there is conflict, both Id and Superego are adamant Ego resorts to defense mechanisms to appease both. We call this as ego mechanisms. Ego mechanisms are a way to deal with the anxiety in a conflict. It tries to minimize the anxiety by resorting to certain defense mechanisms. I will narrate them for a better understanding of the functioning of the mind.

Ego mechanisms

Repression: - What is an unacceptable to our conscious mind is pushed into the unconscious mind. Some Id wishes, impulses and emotions are unacceptable to our Superego and they are pushed to unconscious mind. This is a widely used defense mechanism.

Sublimation: - Here the psychological energy is diverted to achieve a good cause. Here the person will be achieving more like many stalwarts in all fields.

Identification: - Identification with a loved object may ward off his anxiety. It may help him, whereas identification with a wrong object may land him in troubles.

Reaction formation: - Hatred for a person may turn into overt expression of love, e.g.: - A boy sends flowers to his girlfriend after a quarrel.

Displacement: - There is shifting of emotions from one object to another, e.g.: - A mother beats her child after quarrel with her husband.

Rationalization :- The person offers a rational explanation, which may or may not be valid to hide from himself and his actual instinctual motive, e.g.:- he may claim hating a person because he belongs to another religion and actual reason may be something else.

Intellectualization: - It is closely related to rationalization, It refers to excessive intellectual process to avoid painful experience and expression. This is to avoid facing the reality.

Undoing: - It is an attempt to cancel out certain reactions. It is seen in obsessive compulsive neurosis. This is an attempt to undo a forbidden act. e.g.: - when a person gets a murderous or sexual thought, he may try to exonerate himself by saying "leave it" three times.

Denial: - This defense mechanism is widely used in normal as well as pathological states. The degree of its use indicates the severity of the pathology. Excessive denial is seen in psychosis.

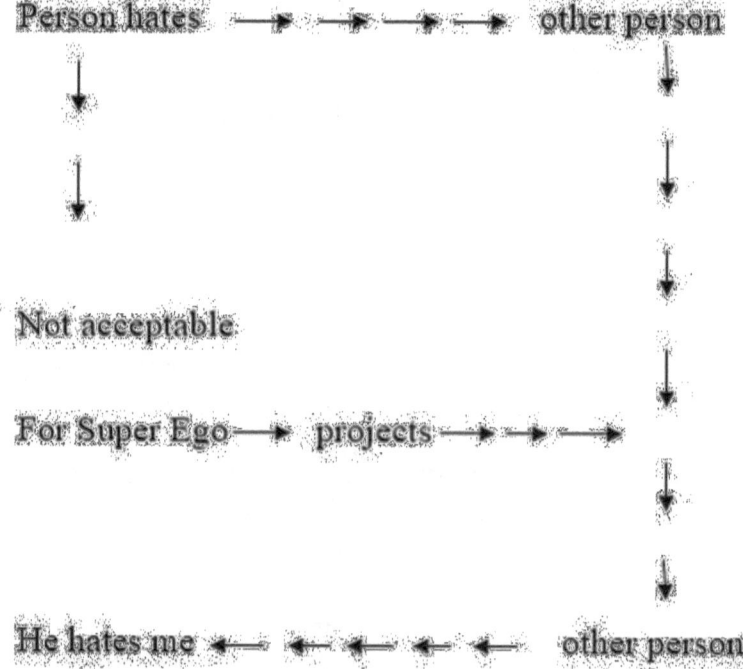

Projection: - A person attributes his own feelings and wishes to another person, because he is not able to tolerate his true feelings, e.g.: - "I hate him" becomes "He hates me". A person hates a person and projects his hate feelings to the other person. It is like projector projecting its picture on to the screen.

Regression: - Here one attempts to revert to an earlier level of development e.g.: - A person who is faced with overwhelming problems of an adult may behave like a child.

Counter phobic mechanism: - The ego attempts to alleviate phobic anxiety by indulging in the same feared activity e.g.: - A person with stage fear may become an orator.

Withdrawal and avoidance: - The ego may attempt to deal with the stress by removing itself from the stressful situation.

All of us use many of these ego defense mechanisms without our knowledge. The presence of these does not mean one is ill. Anything too much is bad, including food and in the same way excessive use of any mechanisms can lead to mental illness. If the defense mechanisms are to the extent of causing severe disturbance in any area of life, that is the criteria for mental illness.

Flower Phobia

Raghav, a 32 years old man came with a complaint of severe anxiety. He had chopped down a tree, which had just begun flowering. He woke up in the middle of the night and chopped the tree. He felt bad for his action. His wife was worried about his action. Raghav was fond of flowers and plants. Being apprehensive about Raghav's chopping of the tree, his wife wanted to bring it to the attention of her father as she didn't know what else to do.

Raghav had completed BA degree and was working in a readymade garment shop. He was a good employee and was liked by the owner. He had received promotions and had become a supervisor. His father had expired 3 years back. His mother had expired when Raghav was 4 years old. His father remarried and had one son and one daughter from the second marriage. His step mother raised Raghav. She was appropriate for the name of step mother. She was not caring for him as well as she cared for her own children. She would shout and beat Raghav at the slightest pretext. At times she had branded Raghav with hot iron and had threatened him not to tell his father. His step brother and sister were not causing any troubles. His father was very busy in work and hardly had time for the family.

As a child Raghav was very upset with his step mother but was helpless to do anything. He used to cry in bed. If he cried in front of stepmother, she would beat him. There were days he could not sleep properly. His father loved him. Once the father noticed Raghav's branded wound and asked him. Raghav told what had happened. His father questioned his step mother. She shouted at Raghav for revealing it. She shouted at her husband and said Raghav touched hot iron accidentally. His father didn't believe it and it ended on a big fight between his father and stepmother. She went and locked inside her room and threatened to commit suicide with an incriminating note on Raghav and her husband. His step mother had even beaten her husband on many occasions. Because of this attitude of step mother Raghav never dared to tell his father any more.

Raghav completed BA degree and then began working in readymade garment shop. While studying in college he met his wife. She was a junior to him in the same college. They used to meet somewhere like park. They decided to marry, and both parents consented to the marriage. Raghav's step brother and step sister went abroad. His father and step mother asked Raghav and his wife to stay with them. His father expired a year later. Raghav was taking care of the family after the death of his father. Raghav, his wife and step mother were at home. Every day his step mother had arguments with him about something or the other. Sometimes they were severe. One day they had a severe argument and in the middle of the night, Raghav chopped sampige tree (a kind of flowering tree with a very nice smell of the flowers) in their yard. It was not a big tree yet. It had just begun flowering.

Raghav was disturbed about his own action. He loved plants and flowers. He puzzled about severity of his actions. His wife was apprehensive about his actions. On examination Raghav had no physical problems. He was anxious and depressed mildly. He was ready to undergo psychotherapy. He had no habits. He had no physical activity. He had no children yet. He got along well with his wife.

Raghav came for the next appointment. He was quite unhappy about his chopping of the tree. He felt that he shouldn't have done it. He again talked of his problem with his step mother. He recalled how she used to beat him and brand him. He expressed how he was unhappy about her. He acknowledged that at least she gave him food. Now he had to care for her. His step mother was a dominating lady and most of the time shouted at him and his wife. He had seen her hitting his father also. Sometimes she threw vessels, etc out of anger.

Even though she was under his care she shouted at him and his wife most of the time. Raghav was of the nature that he should respect elders. As he was not shouting back, his step mother took advantage of it by shouting more. Raghav's wife was a very mild person. Practically his step mother was ruling the family. Raghav hated it, but was unable to express it.

He used to get very angry at his step mother. On the previous day of chopping the tree his step mother had shouted at him. He felt like banging the wall out of anger. He could not get sleep that night. He was so much disturbed that he went and chopped the tree and then was able to sleep. It was clear he took out his anger on the tree. There were other plants and the question was why he picked this tree. Further delving made it clear that this tree was planted by his step mother. She was fond of sampige flowers. After chopping the tree, he slept well as his pent up anger was expressed.

Psychodynamics

Raghav's Child part of the mind (ID) was selfish and hated the partial attitude of step mother. Another part (mature part or EGO) had to tolerate step mother's attitude because of the basic nourishment requirements (survival instinct). This caused conflict in his mind towards her. The adult part of his mind (EGO) had to deal with this conflict. The conflict resulted in aggressive feelings towards step mother. His Conscience (Super ego) hated these aggressive feelings towards step mother as he couldn't go without her for nourishment as a child. This conflict resulted in pushing his unacceptable aggressive feelings to the unconscious mind (Repression). It was only a partial repression as it remained in conscious mind and found expression in disliking her in partial attitude (Mild form of aggressive feelings). A heated argument with his step mother ignited repressed feelings and found expression in conscious mind. The Ego failed to contain it in unconscious mind. It resulted in chopping of the sampige tree.

Here Raghav unconsciously identified sampige flowers with step mother, because she was fond of these flowers. His aggressive feelings were expressed on the tree (displacement). The aggressive feelings on step mother were unacceptable for his superego. It was better to chop the tree than step mother. He was letting out his anger in a more partially acceptable way to his conscience (superego), yet it was not acceptable completely to his conscience, because his act was not normal. As a result of this strong super ego he felt guilty for his action. This resulted in anxiety, depression and phobia.

Psychotherapy

First few sessions were involved in understanding symptoms, life situation, relationships and factors that precipitated the symptoms. The feelings were expressed. Ventilating the feelings calmed him down (it is called catharsis). He was able to understand his problem.

The link between his repressed aggressive feelings on his step mother and chopping of the sampige tree was explored. His step mother was fond of sampige flowers. She had planted the sampige sapling. Raghav's harbored aggressive feelings on his step mother,which found expression in chopping of the sampige tree. In other words his aggressive feelings were to the extent of killing her and instead he chopped (killed)the tree. Why he had to wait till it was about to bloom flowers is a question. Raghav's stepmother was fond of sampige flowers. His aggressive feelings were on the flowers. He hated sampige flowers (step mother) and was afraid of his actions on these about to bloom flowers and hence it was phobia. He didn't want to see the flowers(stepmother).

He felt very unhappy to have lost his real mother. His stepmother did not measure up to his mother. He realized that his expectation was not realistic with step mother. His conflict of Bad mother (stepmother) and good mother (own mother) were realized. Even in bad step mother there was an element of goodness (goodness in bad step mother) that was, she had nourished him. Finally, he accepted his stepmother was not a very bad mother. We can notice the difference in saying bad mother and not a bad mother. An adage every cloud has a silver lining was brought to his notice. Here the dark cloud was stepmother and silver lining was that she nourished him. He accepted it in therapy and decided to love people for their plus points and to ignore their minus points as much as possible.

His feelings and relationship with his stepmother improved. He became more peaceful in his mind. He was advised to involve in some physical activity. The physical activity helps in relaxing the mind also. He was also advised to involve in some activities like recreational, social like meeting people (relatives and friends). He realized in therapy to express feelings as much as possible then and there only, instead of harboring inside. Raghav's case is one of my very interesting cases. The therapy was for nine sessions. He was prescribed anti-depressants and tranquilizers. The medicines were for symptomatic treatment. We are living in a very fast world. People expect to be cured fast. With pharmacotherapy (medicines) psychotherapy process was accentuated

Fear of Death

Kamala, a 30 years old woman came with complaints of uneasiness and anxiety. She had husband with one son and a daughter. They had a car and living in own joint family house. Her husband was good in providing adequately for the family. Her husband would always inform her before taking any important decision. Her in laws were fond of her. If there were any usual quarrels between her and her husband, they were siding towards her. Her husband was adopted son for his parents. Kamala lost her father when she was one year old. She was very fond of her mother. Can anyone think of Kamala having a problem? As per her relatives Kamala had an enviable life.

Kamala had abdominal ache for 6 months. It was diagnosed as appendicitis and was operated. Before surgery her fear of death began. She was afraid that she might die during surgery. Everyone told her there was no need to fear for appendicectomy in modern days. Surgery was over without any problem. She was brought home after recovering from surgery. Fear of death continued in a small way. She would comfort herself that she didn't have any life threatening diseases. In spite of knowing that there was no meaning in her fear and she was not free from it. Five months elapsed after surgery and she knew the threat of any complications from surgery was a remote possibility. Her fear of death continued and gradually increased. For one month it became unbearable.

Being unable to tolerate she decided to see me as she came to the decision it might be psychological. We can appreciate her awareness about psychological problems. Many learned people do not have so much awareness and courage to see a psychiatrist. She was not able to bear her agony and decided to inform her husband. Her husband initially scolded her for thinking it was psychological as she was not mental (his word according to her). Her husband finally agreed and permitted her for psychiatric treatment. He learnt that there was no point in just advising her. He gave permission for psychiatric consultation. After she decided to see a psychiatrist the next problem was whom she should consult. She didn't know any psychiatrist. She was ashamed and scared to ask any doctor because they might label her as mad. Being clever she asked her children's pediatrician that she wanted a psychiatrist for one of her friends. He gave my referral.

Very first thing that she asked me was not to inform the referring doctor. Her husband had been to his work and she came with her lady friend. I sent her friend out and talked to Kamala alone. She was well dressed and if anyone saw her it was difficult to imagine that she could be having any psychological problems. She spoke nicely and had a likable personality. She said the fear of death bothering her too much, otherwise everything was alright. She praised her husband and his family for being good to her. I prescribed her one antianxiety medicine for temporary relief with an advice to see me for further psychotherapy sessions.

I was not aware of her root cause of her fear. This is not uncommon. It will take a while to know. Nobody likes death. Survival is a human instinct. Human being would like to live even with immense problems. How many people calmly take the likely possibility of their death? Even though every one dislikes death, do they fear as much as Kamala? The question was whether she had any worries? The more questions arose than an answer to the problem. Only when the questions arise we may find the answer. No questions means one will never find answer.

In her third visit she accused me that I was thinking that she might be having a desire to die. I had not mentioned it at all, then why she was accusing me? In psychotherapy unconsciously the patient will lead the psychiatrist to the problem. I could have become angry as she was accusing me without a reason. That would have been bad psychotherapy. Here why she was accusing me was more important. To me it meant that she must be entertaining death thoughts. Probably she was leading me to it by accusing me. At that stage it was purely my opinion. I tried to find out from her what I said might have led her to conclude her statement that I felt that way. She was not able to give a reasonable answer.

In her next visit she was smiling in spite of fear. She said that she was angry that I tried to find out the reason. She was hesitant. She said "doctor every family has some or the other troubles, isn't it?". I told her that was true fact of life. Her husband was angry with her. The reason for that became the topic for the next two visits. She said that her husband was a very angry man and would shout for small reasons. House had to be kept clean; if children would have thrown a piece of paper he would become very angry on children and on her. Children should not touch his things. If kamala had kept his things elsewhere, she would have it on that day. In those visits she reported many incidents that made her husband shout. Except for his anger she described him as a good husband. Her husband loved her very much. Because of his anger children were scared to talk to him. She felt bad that children couldn't talk to their father without any fear. Whenever her husband was so angry she entertained death thoughts because she was fed up of his anger. Lately his anger was overwhelming. Underneath the death thoughts she might be entertaining death wishes also (Sigmund Freud said beneath every fear there is a unconscious wish for the same). She readily confirmed it saying husband's anger was the reason for it.

In the mean time her husband had come with her and met me. He said that he didn't know what Kamala's trouble was and ready to do anything on his part. I suggested him that I wanted to see both together for solving some problems. We may call this as marital psychotherapy. In the first joint visit Kamala couldn't bring herself to mention her problem about her husband. She kept talking how good her husband was (may be reaction formation). Again, I saw Kamala separately and asked her why she didn't talk in front of him. She was afraid that he would take her to task for telling all petty things to the doctor. I tried to find out if she was comfortable in talking about the problems in front of him, if I helped her. She said she feared his anger. I said that I would handle it and she agreed to talk in front of him. In such circumstances we must keep in mind husband's reaction and its impact on their future marital life. Only if it was going to be helpful, we should undertake it.

I asked husband to join again. I told him how he would react if something came up in therapy that might not be to his liking. He said that he would take it. I laid down certain ground rules to the therapy session. One should not shout when the other one was talking and should listen without interference. Both will get a chance to present their views. He agreed in front of Kamala. I asked Kamala to present her feelings about him. She was scared. With her permission I initiated by saying the problem was his anger. Her husband raised his voice and I pointed out about our ground rules. Still he was loud and I had to tell him I could not continue that way. He felt sorry and requested me to continue. Kamala mentioned how much she was scared about his shouting. I asked her husband to respond. He admitted that he had problem with his anger. He also didn't like it. He said that he would make efforts to change in expressing his anger. At that point Kamala felt bad that she was letting her husband down by telling all these, which were not in favor of her husband. She felt that she was insulting her husband and felt she was not a good wife. I had to deal with these feelings. Where was the question of letting her husband down because it was revealed only in therapy situation in front of a professional? It would have been letting him down if she had revealed it in front of everyone. Her husband was taken aback how much Kamala was concerned about his reputation with others. He even told her he didn't feel let down and he was happy with her concern about him.

Her husband said that he came up in life with great difficulty. His uncle raised him with discipline. He was punished even for small mistakes. He recognized that disciplined raising was responsible for coming up in life. The discipline was so much ingrained in him; he enforced them on his wife and children unknowingly. He never thought that sometimes a good act like discipline could be a problem also if it was in excess. Even a good thing can be bad if it is in excess. Kamala feared his anger outbursts. She would keep quiet fearing it might end up in a disaster. I made them aware that the situation could have been handled in a better way. Kamala was right in keeping quiet when husband was shouting, but why she didn't try to talk this topic after he cooled down? She agreed and her husband said that he would not stop her from expressing after he had cooled down. This behavior of his shouting and her keeping quiet had become a way of life between them (Eric Berne's Transaction analysis).

Both came to me for follow up after a couple of weeks. Both looked cheerful. Kamala was free from fear of death. A couple of days prior to the visit, children had left toys in the passage obstructing movement. Her husband began shouting and Kamala shouted back saying" I am fed up and you can only put them in proper place if you want" Her husband was taken aback and was surprised at her reaction. Our reaction can also put brakes on others response (action and reaction dictates the final outcome in behavior as per Eric Berne again). It didn't lead to any escalation of the problem as Kamala felt. It boosted her self confidence and it changed the reaction of her husband gradually. Since then her husband was less angry and she was more vocal about his anger. This is a good example of actions and reactions can change the transaction between the two. Our action can potentiate or modify the reaction in other person. As Eric Berne put it what happens between two people is a transaction. Analyzing the transactions leads to a better adjustment. He called this as transaction analysis. Our action can evoke a positive or negative reaction in other person. Kamala's shouting had put a brake on her husband's anger. Another two weeks passed and both of them were cheerful. I suggested them for termination of therapy. Unimaginable her husband wanted to continue therapy saying it had helped them and wanted to understand each other better. I suggested that they could always come back if needed.

Kamala's problem was not madness as people think. She was not able to bear the anger of her husband. She knew it was too much. On the other hand unconsciously, she felt reacting in that situation was unacceptable to her mind. She believed talking back to husband meant that she was disobeying her husband and she was not a good wife. She had inculcated this opinion of the society. It was brought to her notice that talking back in a correct situation was nothing to do being a good or bad wife. This we call it as therapeutic split. Her husband understood and that made the situation better. Psychoneurosis was her problem and it is a highly curable illness. If it is not taken care of in the beginning it may lead to much bigger problems.

Psychodynamics

Kamala had developed a personality nature prevailing in the society i.e, wife is supposed to be loving, passive, obeying and a faithful follower of her husband. Anything contrary was considered as a bad wife. This nature was deeply ingrained in her unconscious mind. In her conscious mind she was not able to bear the excessive anger of her husband. She was a person of patience but the problem was unbearable. The resulting difference between the two parts of the mind caused a psychological conflict. The conflict generated anxiety. She was not able to deal with it and couldn't bear it. When it was unbearable, she wished for her death and this turned into fear of death. According to her unconscious mind it would put an end to the problem. This was not acceptable to the conscious mind because she loved her husband and children. That part of the mind wanted to live. She was torn between the two parts of the mind. Her mind was not able to decide what to do. This led her to seek treatment.

Psychotherapy

In psychotherapy she recognized the problem. She recognized her ingrained personality nature and fear of dealing with the problem. She learnt expressing the right thing was nothing to do with being not respectful to the husband. She came to the opinion that she had to deal with it rather than continuing in the same way. Her change in reaction to her husband's anger brought a change in his reaction towards her and children. Her reaction brought down the anger in her husband. This brought a good homeostasis in the family. Many people in the same category end up in a disaster without seeking treatment. Kamala didn't run away from the problem and decided to face it by seeking help. Her awareness of psychological problems needs to be appreciated. If she had continued the same way without seeking treatment she would have become very depressed and even would have committed suicide. What a disaster it would have been to the whole family. We can recall an adage prevention is better than cure. Kamala prevented a disaster in her family.

Guilt

Mahesh, a 52 years old civil engineer and contractor came to me with guilt feelings. He felt responsible for his daughter's suicide. He was married with one son

His daughter was 21 years old and was studying in 2nd year in medical college. She committed suicide by hanging from a ceiling fan in her room about two weeks before the date of consultation. In fact, she was brought to me about six months before for an opinion. She was too much stressed about her studies. She felt unable to cope up with her studies. She wanted to discontinue her studies in medical college. She was an average student always. She wanted to study medical and her father got her a seat by paying hefty donation. She was alright except for her feeling about her studies. I had advised her to see me for psychodynamic psychotherapy after one week along with a prescription of medicines. She was never brought back to me for follow up. This is very common in our society. The social stigma on mental illness prevents people from seeking treatment.

The above information is important for the readers to understand Mahesh's problem. At first I had to deal with his repentance about the past. I conveyed to him that past had to be put behind. One had to live in the present with an eye on the future. We cannot undo the past. He agreed for this. He felt sorry for not bringing her back to me for further treatment. He knew her problem could have been solved by a psychiatrist; otherwise he would have not brought her to me for opinion. Then the question was what went wrong. His wife and relatives felt her problem was not madness and why she should be treated by a psychiatrist. He partially subscribed for that thinking. A few relatives offered help. Some people advised her not to worry and being an intelligent girl she could complete her MBBS. Some others told her that she should be ashamed to feel like that, when her father had spent so much money for her studies. Yet some others told her parents they should have thrashed her and made her not to feel like that. The above are a few of the responses of close family members. I have not reported all of them. People are very good advisers. Nobody tried to find out why she was not able to cope up with her studies.

Mahesh repented that he listened to others instead of me. This is not uncommon. The social stigma on mental illness makes people vulnerable and shy away from seeking treatment from a psychiatrist. What to do he was also misled by his own well-intentioned relatives, who had stigma on mental problems. Still he continued to say it was a mistake. Even if he considered it as a mistake, did he know anyone who had never made a mistake? To err is human and he agreed that everyone makes mistake. I asked him then why he was hard on himself for the so-called mistake. I asked him if he were to do it all over again, what he would do. He immediately said that he would have brought her to me for treatment. Why there was a difference, because this was an afterthought. Anyone can make the best decision after the incidence is over. Before the incidence even the most intelligent person cannot make the right decision. Life is not without risk. There is an element of risk in everything.

We can classify risks into low, medium and high categories. We must take low and to some extent medium risks always. It is a fact of life. Taking high risk is up to the individual. At the time of taking a decision of not bringing her to me he thought it was low risk. He didn't know the enormity of his daughter's feeling. He was concerned and loved her. Even though she is his daughter, she was a different person. How could he dig into her mind and assess the intensity of her feeling? This was not a mistake or a deliberate act; it was a misjudgment out of ignorance. Nature has given us forgetfulness. All of us hate forgetfulness. We don't understand it is bliss also. If we were to remember all the wrong judgments we have made in our lives, who knows what would happen to us (may be heart attack). Forgetting and forgiving are most important acts in our lives. We have to forget and forgive ourselves first, and then we will learn to forget and forgive others. All these had an impact on Mahesh. He felt relieved. He decided that he had to move on in life. His therapy was achieved in three sessions. He was not given any medicines.

Psychodynamics

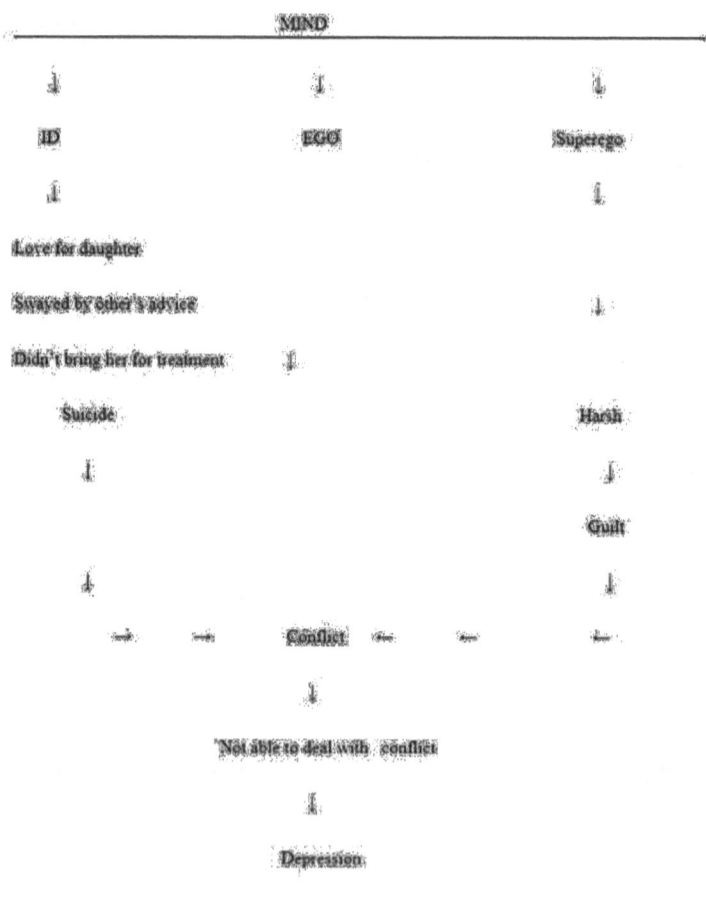

We shall try to understand Mahesh's problem. Guilt is a part of Superego (parent). His superego was harsh. His ID was swayed by well-intentioned relatives. The social stigma and concern about future prospects of her marriage further influenced ego to make the decision of not bringing her to me. The misjudgment ended in suicide. The superego became harsh and guilt resulted. This led to Depression.

Psychotherapy

At first, he was allowed to talk about his daughter's suicide and his guilt. I had asked him if he knew in advance what was going to happen what decision he would have taken. He said certainly he would have brought her to me. Only if we know the result of the future we can avoid all bad decisions. We have to take decisions on what we know at that time. That decision may turn out to be right or wrong, which we will know in future. This is the reality of life. Mahesh's decision turned out to be wrong, but he didn't know at that time. He was too harsh on himself. It was a wrong decision but was not a deliberate act. All these made his superego to accept and be less harsh on himself.

Social Media Addiction

Nandini, aged 21 years was brought to me for consultation on the recommendation of her family physician. The referral letter mentioned that she was suffering from anxiety. She was accompanied by her father. Her father had treatment from me about 25 years ago for depression. Her father mentioned that Nandini's performance in studies had gradually reduced.

I talked to Nandini alone. She mentioned that her performance in studies had reduced. She was a student of 7th semester in bachelor of engineering (BE). She had scored 90% in 10th and 11th standards. Her father got her a payment seat in engineering. She had done well in 4th & 5th semesters of engineering. Her grades began falling in 6th semester and she failed in 2 subjects. She didn't appear even for one subject in 7th semester, because she was not confident about her preparation. She denied any family problem. Her parents got along well. Both the parents loved her and provided all for her necessities. My examination revealed that she had minor anxiety and depression, other than that she was alright. I advised her to see me for psychotherapy sessions.

In the next few sessions many matters had to be dealt. The first thing that came up was that she was lethargic and lazy. She had read in internet that laziness and lethargies could be due to thyroid problem. I ordered thyroid profile and it was quite normal. She was doubtful about the result, saying it could be wrong. I asked her to get her thyroid profile done in a laboratory of her choice and it reported again the same thing that her test results were normal. She accepted it. Then her contention was that she was less intelligent. I had to educate her that intelligence forms in first 5 years of life and later it can improve to a small extent only. Intelligence once formed cannot go just like that, unless there is some kind of brain disease. Her brain was quite normal. Other brain functions like memory, judgment, orientation, etc were normal. She was still not satisfied about not having neurological problem and I asked her to consult a neurologist to clear her doubt. I told her I was sure that she had no brain disease and I suggested her to see a neurologist purely for her satisfaction. The neurologist gave a clean chit that she had no brain disease. Then her question again was that she had less intelligence. She was unable to answer whether she really believed that she was of less intelligence. When she had scored 90% in school how can she be of less intelligence?. At that point she recalled that even in 6th semester she had scored 90% in 2 subjects. How was this possible if she was of less intelligence? To score high marks in any one subject requires high intelligence. She agreed and then she said that her concentration power was gone. I asked her if her concentration was good in any other matter. Her reply was that it was good in face book, internet, etc. I brought it to her notice that in brain there are no different centers for different types of concentration. If her concentration power was bad in studies how it was good for face book, etc. Then she said that her memory was not good. Again she was reminded that her memory was good for face book, etc.

I raised with her that she had thought of thyroid, brain disease, intelligence, memory, etc as causes of her problem and none of them were right. I asked her what else could be the problem?. She said that she had no interest. Interests can be natural and can be acquired. If we didn't like a food in the beginning and continued to eat a few times we will acquire taste or interest for it. This is acquired taste. Here Nandini was not putting effort in studies and she confirmed that. She was not aware of the reason at that point. A psychiatrist must probe the patient's daily routine whenever necessary.

Nandini would go to bed at 10.00 pm and woke up at 9.00 am. After she got up she would check her messages on What's app and then had coffee. She spent daily 5to6 hours on face book, Instagram, what's app, etc. She had no physical activity. She was spending not even 1 hour on studies, because she had no interest. She herself admitted that she spent too much time on social media and she called it as an addiction. At that point it was obvious her involvement in studies was affected by what she called as social media addiction.

She readily accepted her social media addiction and wanted to get out of it and resume her studies. I suggested that very first thing that she had to do was to stop social media involvement. She wanted me to give medicine for that. There are no medicines for everything and some things need a tough decision. She raised an issue that she had no interest and what to do about it. The interest could be developed only by involvement in the subject. The more one gets involved more interesting the subject would be. She was not involved much in her studies. She really wanted to complete her engineering. She was also made to realize that her future will not be good, if she failed to complete engineering. She would have to go for small jobs. She decided to stop social media addiction and involve in studies. That's how the therapy ended. It was accomplished in 5 sessions.

Psychdynamics

Let us look at the psychodynamics of Nandini. All biological instincts are dominated by pain and pleasure principle. Instinctually we tend to avoid pain and seek pleasure. Here Nandini unknowingly was avoiding studies and sought social media. Studies are painful and social media is a pleasure. Always good things are difficult and bad things are easy to cultivate. Good things even though they are painful in the beginning, at a later point will bring a lot of pleasure. The bad things seemingly good in the beginning and later will be very bad for life.

Psychotherapy

In initial few sessions she had to be convinced that she did not have thyroid, neurological illness and other illnesses. Then the question about her intelligence, concentration, memory and interest had to be dealt. After she became aware of her excuses the real reason came out, ie laziness and habituation to social media. She had to be made aware that there was no medicine for curing social media addiction and she had to make a firm decision to quit social media addiction. She was pointed out that she was not good in time management. If she could spend 5 hours on social media the time left for other things including studies was less, because everyone has only 24 hours per day. She decided to stop social media involvement altogether and concentrate on studies.

Examination Fear

Mona, a 14 years old girl studying in 8th standard was brought for consultation. She was repeatedly falling ill just before the examinations. She had abdominal ache, headache, etc, etc. In between the examinations she was perfectly alright.

Mohan was a 19 years old boy studying in PUC was brought with a complaint that his mind would go blank in the examinations. He had prepared well and was intelligent also. The same question paper he could answer very well after the examination.

Ravi a 20 years old young man studying in an engineering college would study late in the night and became drowsy in the examination. His performance was affected.

Swathi a 12 years old girl got frantic about the examination. She feared that she was letting down her parents.

Latha a 14 years old was an easy-going girl. She was procrastinating type. She tried to study a lot in a very short time.

Ranjan 15 years old boy prepared well and tried to review till the last minute of the examination. He got confused.

Namitha prepared well and just before the examination her friend asked if she had studied a chapter. She got anxious as she had not studied that chapter and, in the process, forgot what she had studied also.

What is the problem of all these youngsters? It is examination fear. Examination is a big stress for the students. Nowadays it is even more stressful because of high competitiveness. The examination decides about student's future and it is a test of his competence. When successful it boosts the student's self-confidence. When it is a failure it shatters his self-confidence and it raises doubts about his own intelligence. A failure can lead to a big stress on the whole family, if it leads to a disaster like suicide. If the student scores well and goes to higher education the stress is bound to increase further. A failure or success in the examination influences his standing in the society. The society is highly success oriented and hates failure.

About three months prior to the examination season there is a flood of students with examination related problems in my clinic. This reflects the importance of the examination fear. My intention of this is to share my experience in this with the readers. This is done as preventive medicine. Some of the common queries that I have come across and solutions to them are given below.

1. Intelligence: - one of the common complaints is" I am not intelligent and hence I failed". This is a myth. Most of the people are quite intelligent. Only 4 to5% is less intelligent.

2. Hard work: - Most of the people fail because lack of reasonable hard work.

3. Persistence: - there is an adage, which says" failure is a steppingstone for success". It should be the motto. When an usually successful person faces failure, he introspects and finds where he went wrong. He rectifies his mistakes and succeeds next time. Another person when he fails, he gets discouraged and avoids further attempts. He will remain in failure.

4. Patience: - people have no patience. They want to understand the subject in one reading only. Some difficult topics require repeated studying for understanding.

5. Laziness; - many people are mere lazy and do not put required efforts.

6. Procrastination: - A lot of students postpone their studies. They keep saying they will study from next day.

7. Cramming up: - Some students do not give enough time for studying. They try to study a whole lot in a short time.

8. Time orientation: - everyone has time. Some students are poor organizers of time.

9. Discipline: - we have to have a discipline in our daily routine. Some flexibility may be alright.

10. Peer pressure: - There may be a lot of pressure from peers into antisocial activities.

11. Ragging: - nowadays it has become common. Sometime the ragging is so intense it may cause mental disturbance.

12. Substance abuse: - alcohol and drug abuse has become a big menace. In order to avoid stress the students take refuge in these.

13. Social media habit: - nowadays youngsters are hooked on to mobiles, face book, Instagram, e mail etc.

The parents and teachers should keep the above things in mind in taking care of the youngsters. A good relationship by parents with their children is very helpful in tackling this menace.

Worrying Syndrome

Pushpa, a 62 years old woman consulted me complaining of poor sleep for 4 months. She was married for 40 years. She was a home maker. Her husband had retired from a watch company. They had one son and one daughter. Both were married and well settled in life. Her son was abroad. Her daughter was living in the same city with her own family. Her daughter worked and would leave her child in the care of Pushpa while she was away at work. The son had built a house in which Pushpa and her husband lived. They lived in one portion of the house and another portion was let out on rent.

Her husband was never responsible. He worked regularly and didn't have any bad habits. He was a poor saver. He was poor in managing the finances. He got some pension which was not sufficient for maintenance of the family. The son had allowed them to collect the house rent for their own living expenses and along with the pension they had a comfortable living. Her husband was always irritable, and she had gotten used to that.

At night she would get sleep around 11 pm and woke up usually around 3.30 am. She would have difficulty in falling asleep again. She would do some stretching exercises to get sleep. When she didn't get sleep, she was always worried about something or the other, which were mostly trivial matters for ex: - her husband's elder brother scolded them for being late for some thing about 2 years back.

Her grandchild had breathing difficulty and she slept next to her grandchild and that added to her sleep problem. Her one brother in law died 15 years back and her elder brother died 4 months back.

These were some of the examples of what she ruminated on, when she didn't get sleep. She would ruminate for 1 to 1.5 hours and then again would fall asleep for about 2 hours. Her husband's elder brother had made a threat of physical harm to her husband over a dispute about sharing of ancestral property. She was afraid that her husband's brother might harm her husband as he was a very angry man.

Here two points were obvious. She had sleep problem and she was over worried. As a child she was very sensitive. Even for small matters she would worry too much. Pushpa's mother was an over worrying type of a person also. Pushpa was reluctant to marry her husband but was pressurized into giving consent. Her physical condition was alright.

Psychodynamics

Pushpa had become a worrying natured person. Her mother was also a worrying natured type. Pushpa's identification was with the mother. It was inculcated into her nature as a person and had become a habitual pattern of worrying attitude. This reflected in her sleep pattern. Her feeling not having enough and continuous sleep was disturbing her. She began worrying about sleep and tried to sleep as she expected. Her actions were not conducive. She continued to try to go to sleep unsuccessfully and wouldn't change her approach. The result was continuous mental turmoil. Let us understand her problem in terms of Topographical theory (Ref to mind mystery section). On the one hand (conscious mind) she was not happy with her sleep and on the other hand (unconscious mind) she had a habitual pattern of worrying about sleep. In an illness pain can become a pleasure in a way. According to pain pleasure principle (refer to my mind mystery section) the pain had become pathological pleasure in a habitual manner. This resulted in a conflict between her two parts of the mind (connflict between pain and pleasure). She was not accepting either one of them. The result was anxiety and depression.

Her worrying nature reflected in regard to her brother in law problem also. He had not done any harm to her husband in 30years. Her husband wouldn't leave his claim on the property and she wouldn't leave her expectation of her husband refraining from it. She created conflicts and was not accepting facts in one way or other. We can see her conscious mind was not leaving the fear of threat and unconscious mind could not accept the reality. The result the conflict continuing and generating further anxiety. Pushpa was habituated to worrying and hence she was not accepting things one way or the other.

Psychotherapy

We shall look at her sleep problem. She was getting sleep from 11.00 pm to about 3.30 am and again slept for about 2 hours. This summed up to about 6.5 hours. Most of the people sleep around 6 to 7 hours in a day. The studies show that even 4 hours of sleep is enough. Some of the great leaders of many countries sleep only for about 4 hours at night and are able to function without any problem. Pushpa got 6.5 hours sleep. It was not bad at all, but she was not satisfied and that was an important point. When she wouldn't get sleep, she tried some stretching exercises to fall asleep. Sleep is a natural phenomenon and one shouldn't try to get sleep. Our body will take however much sleep is required. If one gets less sleep it will be compensated the next day by getting more sleep. The more we try to go to sleep the less we will be successful. A lot of people worry about sleep. It is a very big and common problem that we come across daily. In sleep we have deep and light sleep phases. While falling asleep in the night and before we wake up, it is light sleep. Even in our entire sleep period the deep and light sleeps keep on interchanging. After educating her about sleep, her sleep improved to some extent. Gradually she was able to sleep till 6.30 am.

Another problem dealt was her over worrying nature. It was there since her childhood days. This deeply ingrained matter had become a part of her personality pattern and needed more time for improvement. The deeply ingrained matter will perpetually repeat itself always and it becomes like a habit. We call this personality character. All of us have a unique personality character. These personality characteristics often cannot be changed fully. Any reduction of it can be a big help to the patient. She recognized that she had to solve her conflicts one way or the other, instead of keep on worrying.

All of us worry. It can be a normal worry or may be an over worry. Often it is difficult to draw a line between the two. If a worry is causing disturbance like poor sleep, etc. we consider that as over worry. For example, a loss of a small amount of money usually can cause worry for a few minutes. Some people worry for the same thing a few hours or even days also and they are considered as over worriers. Our worries should be reasonable. Some people worry a lot for the loss of a small amount of money. At such times the problem is viewed as very big by the person. This over reaction will have a drain on the body and mind. We should try to accept that loss in the past and see how we can live within remaining amount.

She had a fear that her brother in law might harm her husband physically over the property dispute. The value of her husband's share in the property was about Rs. 20,000.00. She told her husband not to claim that small amount. He wouldn't budge, and he wanted to fight for fairness and lawfulness. The dispute was going on for about 30 years. Even though her brother in law shouted, he had never harmed her husband physically. A person who had not harmed her husband in 30 years is unlikely to be harmful. Of course, one cannot absolutely vouch for it. There is always a risk involved in anything and we must take some reasonable risk in life. She was helpless because her husband was adamant to claim his share. She had no choice but to accept the situation. This was exactly the problem and she kept on worrying and feeling helpless in that situation. She began to realize that there was no point in worrying and to go on as it developed. She agreed what was the point in worrying about something that she couldn't do anything about. Her expectation that her husband should refrain from claiming that amount stopped.

There was another element to Pushpa's problem. There are happy people and unhappy people in every society. What is the difference between the two? The nature has created basically everyone in a similar manner. If we ask anyone to list 10 things on 1 to10 scale what they are happy in their life in one list and what they are not happy in another list, we can be sure that their list of being happy may be one or two points. Their list of being unhappy may be 8 or 9 points. A happy person is happy for the one or two things that he can be happy about and an unhappy person is unhappy for 8or 9 things. For anyone there are more things to be unhappy in his life. It is our mental attitude that can make a vast difference. If we show two people a glass filled with half water and ask for their response? One may say it is half empty and another may say it is half full. Who is correct? Both are technically correct, but there is a difference for a psychiatrist. The first one is a pessimist and the second is an optimist. An unhappy person looks at things pessimistically and a happy person looks at things optimistically. We should learn to look at things optimistically and never loose hopes. The hopes are like fuel to our vehicle. It keeps us going on in life and learning that in psychotherapy she began changing her attitude towards life. With the same life situation, she began to find happiness. She said that there was no point worrying in advance and should take it as it came.

Summary

Pushpa was a very sensitive person ever since her childhood days. She had a less responsible husband. The family property problem added to her worries. Her sleep problem was a result of them and it accentuated her worries. Worrying nature was deeply ingrained into her personality. Her feeling of not having enough and continuous sleep was disturbing her. Her actions of trying to go to sleep were not conducive to fall asleep and wouldn't change her approach. Her financial situation was comfortable, and the children were well settled, in spite of these she was worrying about something or the other. A worrying person will always find something to worry. This had become a habit. In psychotherapy she understood that she was a sensitive and an over worrying person. She realized that she was habitually creating situations to worry and yet hated in another part. She developed insight into her problem. She learnt not to worry in anticipation of pessimistic future. She accepted to never loose hopes in life. It took 7 therapeutic sessions to solve her problem. Her problem is called psychoneurosis. She was given a mild tranquilizer initially to hasten the psychotherapy..

Hypochondriasis

Nagesh a 47 years old man came with history of chest discomfort and palpitations. He was seen by many doctors including specialists. He was prescribed medicines, but his problem was not solved. He had a big list of medications that he was taking. Nagesh was a senior employee in a company. He had a good name. He had a wife and one son. His was a nuclear family. He had a Bachelor of arts (BA) degree.

His problem began about 4 years ago with severe chest discomfort and palpitations. He checked the internet and found out that his symptoms could be a sign of heart attack. He rushed to his physician saying he had a heart attack. The physician examined him and was not able to find any physical problem and declared that he had no heart problem. Anyway, the physician ordered chest x ray, blood test, urine test and ECG and all results were normal. The doctor prescribed him tonics and told him to take rest for a few days. Nagesh went on a vacation with his family for two weeks. He was alright for a few weeks.

After about two months he had a severe headache. Again, he searched the internet and learnt it could be a sign of brain tumor. His physician referred him to a neurologist. The neurologist examined him and ordered for skull x ray, EEG and brain scan. There was no sign of any brain tumor. A few days later Nagesh had weakness in right side of the body and after internet check he thought it was stroke. He went back to the same neurologist saying it must be stroke. The neurologist said that he did not have any stroke. He was satisfied and became alright.

A few weeks later Nagesh had back and leg pains. From internet he felt it could be a sciatic nerve damage with vertebral disc prolapse. He was sent to an orthopedician. The orthopedician examined him and ordered for x ray of his back. There was no sign of any problem.

Nagesh was disillusioned with doctor community for not able to find a solution to his problem. He was lost as to what to do. Nagesh went to meet his friends one day. Casually he told them that he was very unhappy with doctors for not finding solution to his problems. One of them asked what his problem was and Nagesh told him the problems. That friend told him he had a lot of similar problems some time ago and finally it was cured by me. Nagesh took my number and fixed up an appointment.

Nagesh was a well built and was neatly dressed person. He talked fluently. He had brought a big file about his previous treatments. Of course, none of them indicated the presence of any physical illness. He said the doctors were unable to detect his problem. His argument was if he had no illness why he was falling ill again and again. He had confidence in all those doctors and about their professional competence. His contention was the physical illness in initial stages sometimes could escape detection by examination and tests. It was his internet search that was responsible for this half knowledge. He had deeply believed that his illness was in the initial stages and not amenable for examination and tests. My examination did not reveal any physical illness. He asked me if I could detect any physical problem. I told him in the negative. I also told him that human being has body and mind and If we cannot find any cause in the body for the physical symptom then we should look at any psychological causes. He did not accept my words, but ready to try as he had no alternative. He felt bad that I was thinking that he was lying. I told him that he was not lying. I explained to him that mind has different parts; broadly speaking mind has conscious and unconscious parts.

The unconscious mind normally is not amenable for awareness. He said he had read this somewhere, but never thought mind could play such a big role. I prescribed an antianxiety and antidepressant medicines. I advised him to see me for weekly psychotherapy sessions for about 8 to 10 weeks.

In the next sessions he asked if it was a possibility that his illness could be very deep inside and in initial stages. He argued it might have escaped detection either by physical examination or tests. I answered in the affirmative, but I told him it was a very remote possibility in him. He wanted to know why I said it was a remote possibility. Any illness of 4 years duration should have become big and amenable for examination and tests. How could it remain in initial stages for 4 years? Nagesh agreed to this. It meant that he had no physical illness and all doctors were correct.

Still he expressed he might die from the deeply buried illness. People die in seconds, hours and days out of an illness. If his illness was severe why he was living even after 4 years? It meant that he had no illness, which was likely to kill him. He had repeated thoughts of death from illness and was afraid it might become true. He was worried what would happen to his family if he died. In 4 years he had these fears of death for hundreds of times and he was still alive. He was not dying and not leaving his fear of death. If all of our thoughts would become true most of the people would have died by this time. Just because we think of death it won't happen. This counseling had an impact on him.

I told him one should not be afraid of death. Everyone has to die. Only if we knew when and how we would die we could have prevented a lot of problems. Future is uncertain. There is an element of risk in everything. We have to think that we are alright today and hope we will be alright tomorrow also. With this hope only the life goes on. He should not loose hopes and should not worry in anticipation of death.

He was not free of his death fear. Everybody has fear of death sometime or the other. They don't go to the doctors frequently and why Nagesh was seeing the doctors frequently? When a person has fear of death he should see a doctor. When the doctor rules out any illness he should accept it and be happy. Why Nagesh was still preoccupied about his death? For everything there must be a reason. I had to probe further. Behind every fear there is an unconscious wish(Sigmund Freud). We fear our own hidden wishes. With this in mind I asked Nagesh any stresses he had. He began saying he had some issues with his boss. The boss was giving him more and more work. Sometimes he felt like resigning from work, but he had no other income to fall back on. At those times he had fear of death. Nagesh was the type of person who would finish that day's work on that day itself. As Nagesh was finishing all the work given to him in time his boss continued to give him more and more work. It had become almost impossible for him to finish all the work that he was given lately. I asked Nagesh if he ever talked to his boss about this and he never did.

I tried to find out why he did not talk to the boss. He said that he respected his superior and it was his duty to obey him. We can feel the conflict here. He could not bear very heavy work and yet he could not say it as the boss was elder to him. Nagesh said he was given more work than others of a similar position. Always his boss had given a good rating on Nagesh every year. It meant he was liked by his boss. Then why was this problem? Nagesh was mild mannered and obedient person. This is a good example of anything too much is bad also. The next question before me was how to solve this. Nagesh was not prepared to talk to his boss frankly as he was too scared. I asked him if there were any days he had not finished the assigned work and gone for the day and what was the reaction of his boss? His boss did not say anything. I told Nagesh there are two types of communications viz:- verbal and non verbal communications. We can communicate "no" without verbally saying "no". I told him that Nagesh was finishing all the work assigned to him and hence he was shoved with more work. It was a government organization. Other fellow workers were militant type and refused to do even medium work. The boss was under pressure from the top to get the work done. In such circumstances people like Nagesh become victims. One has to work but doing over work continuously is harmful. I suggested Nagesh to do the reasonable quantity of work for the day and to keep the rest of the work pending. When the boss asked him next day he could say that he would finish on that day. When he kept it pending for a few days the boss started giving him about 10 to 15% less work. The problem was solved.

Psychodynamics

Let us look into the psychodynamics here. Nagesh was a very mild mannered, obedient and a good worker. In a government organization only, a few people work, and the boss gives them more work for those who do work. The boss may know it is wrong, but he has the pressure to get things done. The additional work Nagesh had to bear was taking a toll on his health. He was not the type to evade the work and kept finishing it. It was going beyond his limit. At that time he developed fear of death. A person can die of suicide, illness and accident. People have tried to die by going in front of a bus and the driver avoids it by putting brakes. It is not in the hands of the person completely. It is not easy to commit suicide as people say. It requires a great deal of courage to carry it out. Nagesh did not have the courage. The only acceptable choice was illness. If illness could kill him and it saved him from blaming himself for the death.

A person who has death wishes will choose a serious disease, which is likely to cause death like heart attack, etc.

Psychotherapy

One of my professors, John Dorsey used to say psychotherapy was like peeling an onion. In onion we peel outermost layer first and it leads to the next layer. If we keep on peeling layer by layer ultimately, we come to core of the onion. In psychotherapy understanding from most outer mind (conscious mind) presenting symptoms to reaching inner core (Unconscious mind) layer by layer was achieved.

Heart problem, Brain tumour, stroke, etc.
↓
Death fear
↓
Unconscious wish for death
↓
Excessive pressure at work
↓
Obedient nature
↓
Not able to say "NO"
↓
Understood to communicate "NO" without saying "NO"

In psychotherapy it was brought to his awareness that he had repeated physical symptoms, which had no basis in the body pathology. It was brought to his awareness that some physical symptoms could be caused by mind also. He was educated in regard to the presence of divisions in the mind. The reason could have been in deeply hidden in the unconscious part of the mind. The topic of death was discussed as above. His overbearing work could be the reason for his death wishes. The problem of being too obedient and unable to say "NO" even for a good reason was dealt with. He was also told that one could communicate "NO" without saying "NO". He began implementing to communicate" NO" without saying "NO". His problem was solved. It took six psychotherapy sessions to solve his problem

Sun Allergy

Sun rays are essential for light and for living. We cannot imagine the world without sun. Is there anyone not able to tolerate the sun light? Sun's allergy is unimaginable and against nature. One girl was brought to me with sun allergy.

Shobha was a 15 years old girl. Her age was such that she should have been full of energy. Her parents brought her to me saying she had sun allergy. She was already seen by some specialists, who had ruled out all physical illnesses. Allergist said it was sun allergy and treated her without any improvement. At the end he said that she might be having some psychological problem that could be responsible for her allergy. Allergy can be caused by psychological problems also. Shobha's parents were angry at the allergist because of his opinion, they construed that he was suggesting that she was mad. According to them she was not mad at all. They refused to take her to a psychiatrist. So allergist conducted some more tests and gave further treatment and it didn't help. He finally told them to consult a psychiatrist again. Her parents were angry and consulted another Allergist. After all the examinations and treatment he also suggested them to consult a psychiatrist. Her parents cursed the whole doctor community out of frustration. Their contention was they were caring for her in all possible ways and how a 15 years old girl could have psychological problems. She was their only child and parents loved her a lot.

Being disillusioned by the allopathic doctors they consulted ayurvedic, unani etc doctors Meanwhile they performed worships and sought the help of a Mantravadi (person who claims that he can cure illnesses by chanting spiritual mantras). Shobha's illness got worsened. Out of sheer helplessness they decided to bring her to me.

Shobha's parents were very worried. Who would not be worried?, when it happens to their only child. Parents cried in front of me. I had to console them. They had left hopes. I told them not to lose hopes. They said probably there was no cure for Shobha's illness. We are living in 21st century and there must be some cure for her problem. Any way they were ready to try psychiatric treatment out of desperation. Shobha's problem began about 6 months ago. It had worsened lately. The moment sun rays fell on her there were small rashes on the skin with severe itching. It was unbearable for her and it was an agony for them to see her at that time. If she continued to expose to the sun she would have giddiness and would even fall unconscious as per the parents. If she was kept in a dark room there was no problem at all. She stopped going to school because of this problem and stopped coming out of her room. They had covered her room windows with thick cloth sheets to prevent sun rays coming into the room. Shobha came fully covered with clothes in order to prevent exposure to sun rays. Only eyes, nose and mouth were not covered. She spoke slowly. She expressed sadness at her problem and felt fed up. She entertained death wishes but wanted to live for the sake of her loving parents. Her higher mental functions were alright. She had some depression and anxiety. There was no psychosis. Her sensorium was clear. I prescribed an antidepressant and an antianxiety medicines and asked her to come next day.

She was brought to the appointment on the next day by her parents. I saw Shobha alone. She was very talkative, and her grasping power was excellent. She was a topper in school. Her father was a government worker with low salary. They had a small house. The parents got along very well. Theirs was a middle-class family.

Her grandmother lived with them. Her grandfather had expired some years ago. She was very fond of her grandmother. In school she was liked by teachers and her classmates. There were no problems for her in school and from classmates. She had no physical problems. I asked her if she was worried about anything. She denied it. The TAT test revealed that she had some fear about some sexual matter. She was asked to come the next day.

She greeted me saying "good morning uncle". She was a friendly person and had already felt at ease with me. We don't generally indulge in talking about the problems immediately. She said that she had a good sleep. She noticed that she was getting up a little earlier than before. She felt disturbed about her problem. She had no problem in exposing to the sun rays before and why she had the problem now. She felt lost and entertained death wishes. She would have not minded dying if she didn't have such loving parents. She had lost hopes. I told her not to lose hopes. There must be solution for everything. We had to be patient and optimistic.

She had seen many doctors including specialists with no solution for her problem. She had not seen a psychiatrist before. Even though she was advised to see a psychiatrist, her parents were not for it. She had no opinion of her own. Whatever her parents decided she was ready to accept. She was not an adult and it was appropriate for her age to fall back on parent's decision.. She had not yet developed confidence that her illness could be cured by me. There was no improvement and it was her fourth visit. Her problems kept increasing and her parent's anxiety was increasing. I decided to perform a narcoanalysis examination.

The narcoanalysis was done in a nursing home. It is also called as narco test and truth serum test. It is done widely by criminologists to find out the truth from a criminal. Here I never thought Shobha was lying at all. Here it was necessary to hasten the process of the treatment as the parents and Shobha were getting frustrated. I wanted to explore her unconscious mind. A patient may not be lying and hiding a truth deliberately. The problem may have been pushed into the unconscious mind, because it is very painful for the conscious mind. All these happens unawaringly. In this examination we inject a medicine to make the patient lose control over her conscious mind and then the unconscious mind comes out without any checks.

The narcoanalysis was very helpful in Shobha. The summary of the revelation was quite interesting. The arrangement in sleeping was that her parents slept in one room and she shared the room with her grandmother. In the neighborhood there was a man. In the dawn of some days he would come to their room and slept next to her grandmother. There was some faint talk between them, and she would hear some sounds from there. She was not aware of what was going on. She was disturbed about it. She sensed that it was something not normal, but she didn't know what was going on. After some days when she heard some sounds from them, she became disturbed more and curious also. She began to be awake and act as though she was sleeping to hear their sounds. This became a usual pattern. After a few days she realized something of the type that goes on in movies was happening between her grandmother and that man. Gradually she hated what was going on between them. She felt bad about her grandmother. She thought of telling her parents. What to say to parents, because she didn't know what was going on. She was not able to disclose and not able to bear it also. A conflict was created in her mind. That incidence between grandmother and that man was happening in the dawns. She hated it. Her mind associated dawn to that incident. The result was that hate on the incidence was displaced on to dawn. This transformed to allergy to dawn. Shobha couldn't avoid dawns and hence couldn't avoid allergy.

Shobha was eager to know the result of her narcoanalysis. When I revealed that what was going on between her grandmother and that man was responsible for her allergic problem. She said that she was disturbed about it and didn't know what to do about it. She knew what was going on between the grandmother and that man was not natural, but she didn't know explicitly. My next problem was how to solve this problem. I suggested Shobha to get up when that man came in the dawn and that would discourage them. She was scared to do it. She was afraid that her grandmother might become angry.

It was a brainstorming situation to me also. If I revealed it might be a disaster. If I didn't reveal the problem would get worsened. My inclination was to tackle it with least disturbance to the family. I decided to talk to her grandmother without revealing the matter to anybody else. I asked her grandmother what was going on between her and that man. Of course she denied it initially. I told her it had a very bad effect on Shobha. She finally broke down and agreed that there was a relationship between the two. She cried saying that she lost her husband a long ago and the sexual deprivation led her to this. She promised that she would put an end to it and requested me not to reveal it to anybody else.

After a month Shobha and parents came. They expressed immense gratitude to me. Shobha was free of her sun allergy. She was able to go to school as before. Her parents were not aware how her problem was solved. They tried to know from me the reason and I avoided telling them. According to them it was a bad time for them and it cleared because that bad time had passed. They even said that their worships yielded late results.

If I had revealed the truth to thwart their ignorance the whole family's homeostasis would have been disturbed and who knows what would have been the ending. We have taken Hippocrates oath and we have to act in the interest of the whole family. What all mattered was to cure Shobha's problem. Why I should worry about the ignorance of her parents in this issue?. Goldsmith has said ignorance is a bliss some times and definitely it was a bliss in this case.

Psychodynamics

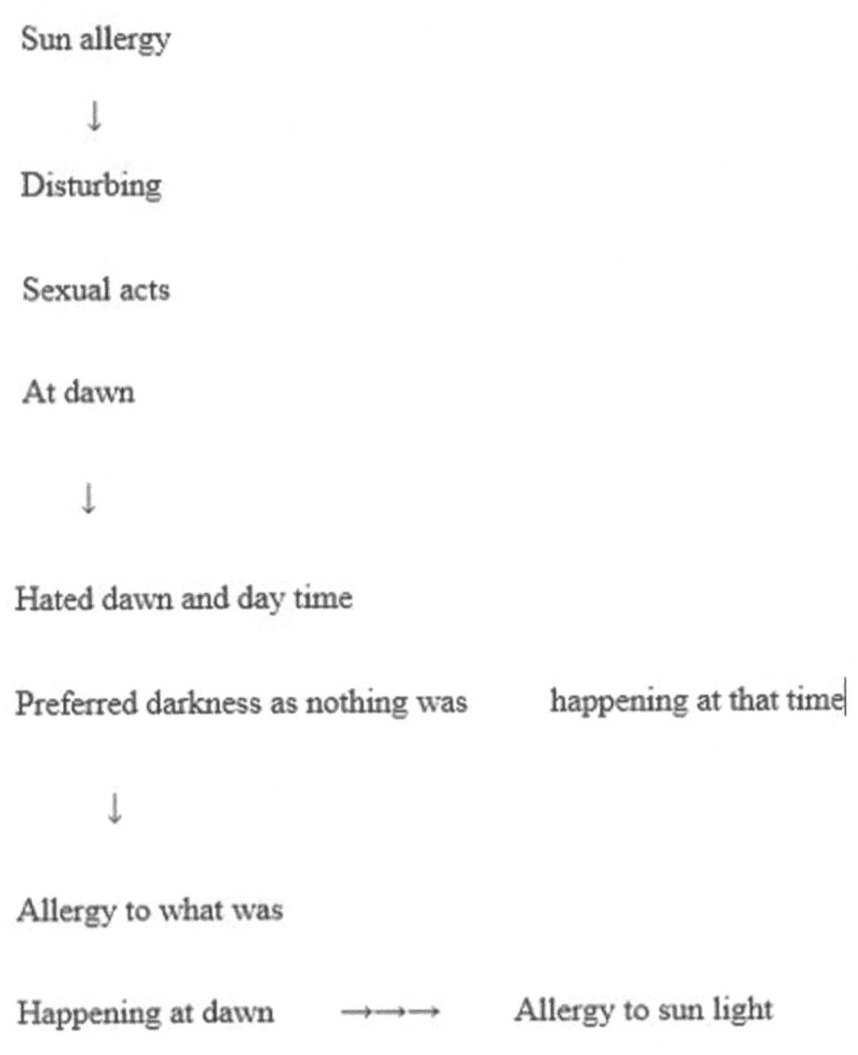

Sun allergy

↓

Disturbing

Sexual acts

At dawn

↓

Hated dawn and day time

Preferred darkness as nothing was   happening at that time

↓

Allergy to what was

Happening at dawn →→→ Allergy to sun light

Psychotherapy

The problem was solved with no disturbance to the family. If I had revealed the family,it would have faced a lot of disturbance in homeostasis. It could have a very serious repercussion on the whole family. What effect it would have on Shobha and her parents was unimaginable. Revealing the truth to them would have changed their interpersonal relationships. It could have a worst impact on the whole family. The problem was solved without the awareness of Shobha and her parents. We as doctors have taken Hippocrates oath. Our actions should be in the interest of everybody concerned. I am happy that I have achieved that.

Inferiority Complex

When a 30 years old male Jagadish wanted to see a psychiatrist, all were surprised. He had a well-paying job and his wife had a good job also. They had a cute small one-year old son. None of them had any illnesses. It was envying type of a life for some. When a person like this wanted his acquaintances to suggest a psychiatrist, all were surprised. He told them that he wanted it for his friend and got away.

Jagadish came inside breathing hard. I wondered whether he had heart attack at first. I told him to relax and there was no need to be in a hurry. He said, "doctor I feel ashamed to say what is in my mind". Jagadish had already consulted a physician and he had given a clean chit to him about any physical illness. He was not peaceful in his mind at any time. He had difficulty in mingling with people. At work if anyone asked something, he had difficulty in answering. Even if he was right, he could not justify it. If superior officers asked something, he was afraid to answer. Even if he knew the answer, he had difficulty in expressing anything. Later he would feel bad for not giving answer. He would feel that he was stupid. He began feeling like this at the age of 14 years. It was on a very minor scale. Lately it had increased. He had not revealed this to anyone including his wife. Sometimes he felt so bad about this that he felt he should have not been born at all. He loved his wife and son of one and half years. Because of them he wanted to live. He couldn't watch even TV because of his restlessness. He couldn't go out much. For everything he had anxiety. He was not even getting good sleep. He had headache in the posterior part of his head. It was frequent and sometimes very severe. He would squeeze his head tight as he was not able to tolerate the headache. He often tied a cloth around his head tightly to get some relief from the headache. Sometimes he had abdominal ache also. The doctor diagnosed it as gastritis and advised him to avoid spicy and sour foods.

Jagadish was a shy and aloof person. Some people talk with ease even though they be afraid. He said, "sir I am afraid to talk to you because you may say I am mad". This is the reaction of most of our patients in the initial stages. He was able to express this much, which was a good sign. I assured him that his problem was not at all madness as he felt. If he was mad (as he thought) how he has achieved all the things in his life. This made him more comfortable. Jagadish was quite inhibited and often would hold his hands tight out of anxiety. When I asked if he was afraid, he replied affirmatively. TAT examination revealed that he had inferiority complex. I advised him for psychotherapy and prescribed some antianxiety agents.

In the next week he came for the scheduled appointment. He said that he was better, but he looked very tense. I told him that he didn't look better to me, and he agreed. 14 years trouble could not be solved in one week. Then the question was why he said that he was better. He was afraid that I might become angry if he said he was not better. This indicated that he would even mask the truth in order to impress other people. A patient should always tell exactly what he felt and then only a doctor can give him the right treatment. Any cure needs a lot of time particularly psychiatric problems. Sometimes we may have to increase the medicines, some other time we may have to change medicines. Some medicine work well in some people and some other medicine works well in others. Pharmacotherapy is an art also. This was only second visit and I had initiated the psychotherapy. We must observe patient's thoughts and actions carefully. His natural characteristics are bound to repeat in therapeutic situation. If we understand them, we will be able to solve the problem.

Jagadish would even tell a lie to impress others. He was doing that with everyone. He enjoyed when they were impressed with him when he lied. Is it wrong? not at all. All of us want to please others, but most of the people do not go to the extent of lying to please others. This was more than usual in him. Jagadish also agreed he was over doing it. Even at work he was telling lies to make it look better. Sometimes the higher officers caught him lying and they were angry with him. In other words what he was trying to achieve by a lie, was exactly the opposite he was getting. People always say they got opposite of what they wanted and blame fate for it. Is it really fate or is it our unconscious mind that will drag us to where we belong? It is our unconscious mind that drags us to the point and people blame fate for it.

In the next visit Jagadish was a little cheerful. He said however much he tried to tell as it was, still he was not able to. Many years of habit or nature cannot go that soon. When a person tries to change sooner or later, he succeeds. Here it was good to know that he was trying. This was a progress in therapy. When I appreciated this, he was taken aback. He was used to curse himself as a useless person. In the following visit he reported that for the first time he felt good for telling something as it was and without telling a lie. He was not good in making friends. He felt that he envied people who were good in getting things their way and felt bad that he didn't have that nature. When he came across such people, he would feel jealous. He dreamt of becoming a big officer but doubted whether he could manage it. Even though he was daydreaming of becoming big it didn't interfere in his work and he got promotions. If he didn't daydream too much and worked better probably, he might have gotten more promotions.

In the next three visits he repeatedly talked of the same things. He had not talked much about his wife's job and her earnings. I had not enquired about his or his wife's earnings. Some people do not like to reveal their income. It is considered as personal. Usually we never ask about their income. Sometimes we must wait for a long time for the patient to talk about incomes, if it is relevant for the therapy then only we discuss. At last he mentioned that his wife's earnings were more, and he looked at my face as if I might say something. I didn't react. This spontaneous revelation must be significant. His mind was trying to drag me to this matter. He repeated that his wife's earnings were about two times more than his earnings. I asked him if he had some feelings about it. He denied and said it came to his mind and he revealed it. Without even asking he had brought up this matter and denied having any feelings about it. At that point I recalled that he felt that he was not as good as some others and whether it had some connection to his wife's earnings. When I brought this matter him again if he had some feelings about it, he admitted positively. We can sense his inferiority feelings here. In our society there is a feeling that a man should have better earnings than his wife. A man doesn't want to marry a woman with higher education and higher earnings. Jagadish's wife was higher on both aspects. His daydreaming to be a higher officer could be the reason to satisfy his masculine pride. Because he was not able to achieve it perhaps he felt inferior. I want to say here to my readers these were just the observations in my mind about his problem.

I had to wait to see if it was right or wrong. The time would tell always. In the next visit Jagadish said that people made fun of him as he was getting less income than his wife. In his wife's job there were a lot of senior people and they retired. She got promotions faster. Jagadish was not that lucky in it. Because both were working Jagadish had to help his wife in household chores also. Sometimes he was doing more work than his wife. Sometimes if his wife was lazy, he couldn't scold her even though he felt like it. He was afraid his wife might get angry and say that she earned more than him. It was only his feeling and his wife not even once expressed like that.

After talking so much about his wife earning, he admitted for the first time it bothered him. I want to point out he had talked about his wife earning more, but always he denied it bothered him before. Many men have married a higher educated and higher earning wife and still quite happy. Then why Jagadish was not? He had accepted and married outwardly and internally (unconsciously) not accepted it. This was the conflict and he agreed. Our mind can be compared to a boxing fight. When two boxers fight the stronger one will win. In a conflict of the mind the stronger part will win. Here in Jagadish it was alright for conscious mind for his wife's higher earnings, his unconscious mind had not accepted it. The unconscious mind was strong enough to keep on giving trouble. Here Jagadish had not come to terms within himself about his wife's earnings. The marriage is between a man and a woman. It is not between two degrees or money. He was mixing up the two and he agreed. All these counseling had better impact on Jagadish. I said it was purely his feeling because his wife never even once expressed it. She was even giving all her salary to him and requested him for money for her requirements. This was the mistake on his part. If a wife earns more does it mean she is better? (therapeutic split as we say). Only, he had felt it. Isn't it these are some of the feelings in our society? They were husband and wife, but he had brought education and earnings to the marriage.

Gradually his relationship with wife improved. He admired his wife for being a very good wife to him. He stopped feeling inferior to his wife. He had inferiority feelings in other areas also. Inferiority feelings may become intense when a person gets a very big setback in life. This may be temporary. In Jagadish's case it was not because of any set back. It was built into his natural personality. Our personality begins to develop from childhood itself. His father was very strict in raising the children. He had a high ambition on children. He wanted children to excel in life. He would point at better studying children and tell him to be like them. The comparison nature was ingrained.

Jagadish wanted to please his father by studying well. He couldn't measure up to his father's satisfaction. He began developing inferiority complex. He was a good student but not enough to please his father. This caused inferiority feelings in him. Jagadish was one of the top few students, but not a topper. I asked Jagadish how many people can be toppers? He said only one can be a topper. Did it mean others were inferior? He couldn't respond to it. I asked if one couldn't get a rank what is wrong in getting first class. He agreed. First class might be less than a rank but not inferior. There is rich class and there is poor class. In between there is a medium class. What is wrong in medium class? These discussions had an impact on him. We should try to achieve higher and when we cannot get it, we should settle for less. This is the truth of life. We tend to compare ourselves with those who are better than us. There are a whole lot of people who are not better than us. We should not look down upon them of course, but we should feel satisfied that we are not that bad in our situation. We should try hard for achieving more and finally settle for what we get. My psychotherapy had a big impact on him. He began to look at his wife as wife only and nothing else. He began to be what he was rather than trying to make better impressions. He felt that he was so peaceful in his mind. The therapy was terminated.

We can label his problem as neurosis. Neurosis is the result of conflict between conscious and unconscious minds. It cannot be treated by just medicines alone. It may give some immediate relief and patient is going to be back again and again. Exploring his deep-rooted conflict is the only way for a permanent cure.

Psychodynamics

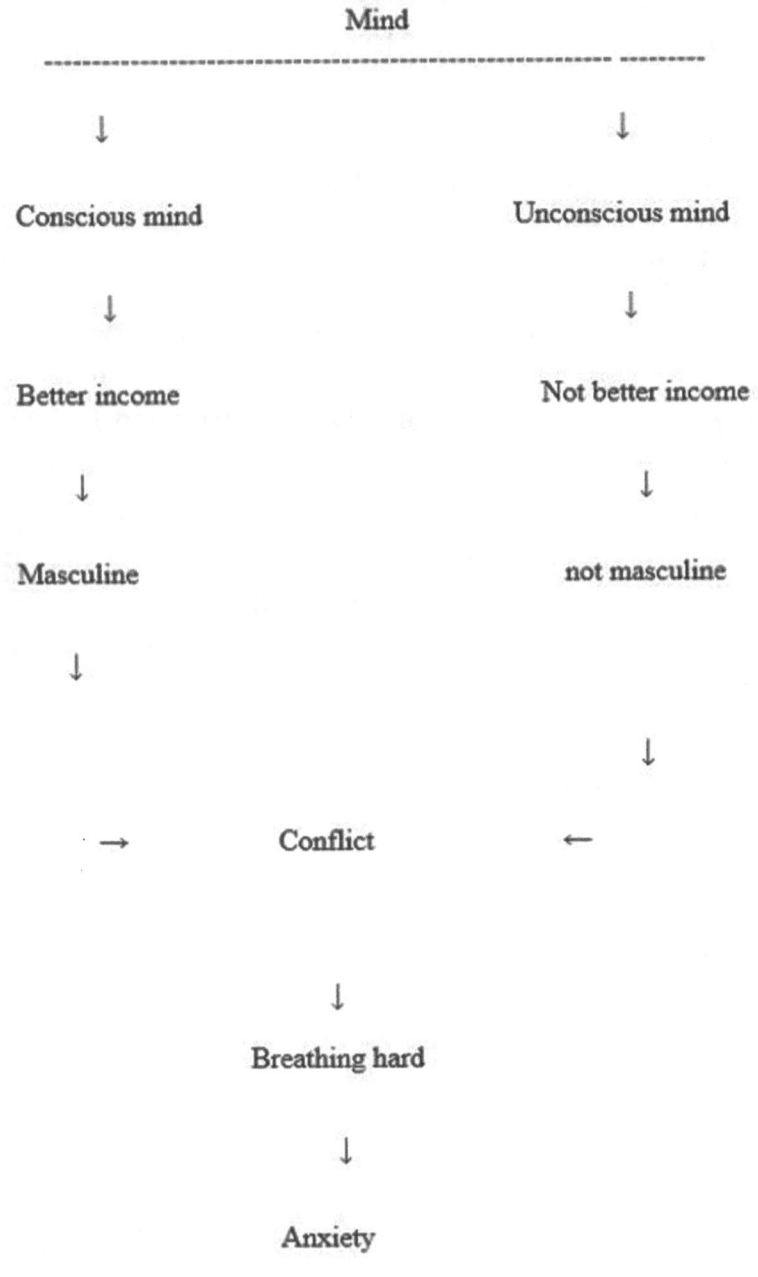

As a child he had developed inferiority complex. It was to do with his father. His desire to earn more reignited his inferiority complex. He was guarding his relationship with his wife that she might talk back saying that she earned more. She never did that, but he continued to feel like that because of his inferiority complex. He was comparing too much about incomes. This resulted in anxiety and breathlessness.

Psychotherapy

Initially it was brought to his awareness that his somatic symptoms had a deep root in mind. The existence of conscious and unconscious minds was revealed. He became aware that he had feelings about incomes of his and his wife. He felt less than his wife, because she earned more. This affected his masculine feelings and felt inferior. He couldn't accept it or reject it. The resulting conflict was explored. This inferiority feeling was deep rooted and was in relation to his upbringing. He realized that marriage was between a man and a woman. He was bringing other factors like money into it. He became aware that too much comparison was wrong. He began looking at his wife as wife and nothing else. The awareness of the conflict brought homeostasis in his mind.

Poor Concentration

Raju, a 13 years old boy was brought to me by his mother for his poor concentration. He was studying in 7th standard in a well reputed private school. He was always a good student and was one of the top-level students in his class till 6th standard. He had been an obedient boy.

His parents were non consanguineous, and the delivery was normal without any complications. His developmental milestones were normal. Physically he had no problems. Theirs was a rich family and parents got along well. He had a younger brother of 11 years old and normal in all respects. Parents were healthy physically.

The above information was adequate for me to proceed further. I asked the mother to sit outside and talked to Raju alone. He was scared. On probing further I came to know he was afraid that I would give him pricks. I assured him that I just wanted to talk to him, and I would not give him a prick. He was in extreme fear and was eager to get out of my chamber. When I asked a question either he would not respond or would respond in one word. He was uncomfortable. My next task was how to make him comfortable with me. Instead of asking about his problem, I began asking him about his interests. I found out he had a fascination for cricket. He was a fan of Sachin Tendulkar. We spent the whole session talking about cricket. Readers might think that what I was doing by talking on cricket. I would say whole heartedly it was not a waste of time. Sometimes a psychiatrist must talk about other things in order to establish a rapport with the patient. The first session ended that way.

In the next session I greeted him saying how was the fan of Sachin Tendulkar ?. He spoke to me with a smile for the first time and said"OK uncle". This showed I had established a workable relationship. Again, after talking about cricket I enquired about his friends and school. By that time, I noticed that he was quite comfortable with me. When I enquired about his studies, he was hesitant. I told him I was not there to take any actions on him, and I was there to help him in his studies. This gave him confidence and he began opening about his problems. His first reaction was that he had poor concentration. He would just sit in front of the books and his mind wandered. He tried hard with no avail. He felt very bad. He could not say what was wrong. He agreed that his concentration was good for cricket. He was lost as to the reason why his concentration was not good for studies. Both parents wanted him to score well in examinations and he wanted it also. Parents had provided all the necessities for him to study. They had arranged private tuition also. He had to get up at 7 am and had to get ready to go to school by 8.15 am. He would return from school by about 4 pm. He would take some snacks and milk and had to run for private tuition by 5 pm. He would come back from tuition by 7 pm. Then he had to do his homework and study till 9 pm. Then he took supper and went to bed. I was appalled by his very busy schedule.

Raju was an intelligent boy and I wondered whether he needed such a hectic schedule. I tried to find out how was his concentration on Sundays and holidays. He said that his concentration was much better on those days. For the first time it occurred to me that he might have been overburdened. He had no time to play on weekdays. His mother made him sit for study at the set study time. He was exhausted and couldn't concentrate. I asked Raju whether he was eager to try something different. He was ready to try. I asked whether he felt that he needed that much private tuition. He did not feel it

Poor Concentration

was necessary. He wanted some time for play also. I ascertained from him that whether he was eager to produce good results if he was given time for play. He enthusiastically agreed.

I had a session with his mother and asked her why she had made it mandatory for him to have private tuition. She was of opinion that Raju was intelligent and with private tuition he would excel. I asked her whether that purpose was being achieved. She admitted it was not. Then I asked her whether she was ready to try a different method. She was scared. The present method was not working and why not try a new method. She asked me whether the new method would work. I told her that I could not assure her of that. The present method was 100% failure. At least a different method had 50% possibility. She agreed to try. I suggested her to have private tuition for only when Raju had difficulty in something, like problem-oriented teaching. Meanwhile Raju was very eager for this.

His mother told me that his teacher refused for this arrangement as it resulted in some monetary loss to him. She was lost as to what to do. I suggested her to tell the teacher that she would pay the same existing fee, but her son will approach the teacher only whenever the problem arose. The teacher agreed for this and even told her that he could take one more student. This showed the greediness of that teacher. Anyway, this was beside the point. With this arrangement I suggested his mother to bring him to me once a month for follow up. There was an internal test and Raju was back in the top few in the class. I suggested Raju to be brought for follow up once in 3 months till the final examination. He was brought to me after receiving the final marks card. He had surpassed others and was number one in the class. His mother thanked me saying I was god to them. I said that I had done my duty as a doctor.

In this case we have to look at the family psychodynamics rather than Raju's alone, after all he was a minor. His father was a busy businessman and mother took care of all family matters. His mother was strict and had high ambitions on her children. She wanted the best of Raju in studies. She had disciplined him and had set up his study time. Raju was an obedient and mild -mannered boy. He had a very busy schedule with no time to play. We can recall an adage "All study and no play made Jack a dull boy". Raju would faithfully follow whatever mother imposed, but his mind wouldn't listen. The result was he could not concentrate. This is a good example of anything too much is too bad, even a good one. The high expectation of parents can cause problems to the children. Another important lesson in life is when one method is not working, try another method. Raju was not given any medicines.

Narrow Mindedness

Niranjan 28 yrs. and Latha 26 yrs. came to me for consultation. One of my previous patients had referred them to me. Niranjan said that Latha had been unhappy with poor sleep and bad mood. He couldn't understand why she was like that. Many times, he had asked her as to why she was like that. She always said that she was happy. Niranjan loved her and he knew that she loved him also. His parents and only younger sister also loved his wife. All of them got along very well. Financially the family was of upper middle class and quite comfortable. It was an arranged marriage, but with mutual consent. The physical examination didn't reveal any illness. Niranjan was lost as to what to do. At that time, he came across with an old patient of mine, who suggested him to see me.

I saw Latha privately for confidential reasons. I have observed in general the patient feels more comfortable in sharing the intricate matters to the unrelated and nonjudgmental professional. If at all it is revealed in front of the loved ones there will be inhibition and/or over reaction out of love and matters get worsened. In my experience I have seen patients reveal a lot privately to the doctor. Some things people cannot express in presence of another person because of inhibitions. I assured Latha of confidentiality and to express anything and everything without any hesitation. She totally agreed with what Niranjan had said. She was very happy with Niranjan, his parents and his sister. They loved her and didn't give any troubles. Her husband was good, responsible and loving. She said that she was happy in the marriage. He would take her out to movies, parks, restaurants, etc,

etc. She agreed that she was unhappy and unable to point out what it was about. Her parents loved her, and everything was alright there also. We had reached a roadblock about her problems.

In the next visit I told Latha that there must be something she was unhappy and to tell me even if it was a very small matter. She requested me not to feel bad about and it was a very silly matter (She described it as silly). I encouraged her to tell me and assured her that I would not make any judgment like that. She told me that her husband is close to a 15 yrs. old girl. She had also met that girl along with husband. That girl is also a nice girl, by name Meena. Meena called patient's husband every day and sometimes they met in her school for a cup of coffee. They were like brother and sister. Meena was so close to Latah's husband that she had discussed with him certain things that even her parents didn't know. Latha didn't like their relationship. She had full confidence in her husband, yet she couldn't accept it. She felt that she was a very narrow-minded person to think like that about her loving husband. She felt guilty for having entertained such thoughts about their relationship. She, herself couldn't voice this to her husband. She talked to her mother about this and she scolded her for her narrow mindedness. Her mother told Niranjan was a very good person and had high confidence in him that he would never do such a thing; after all theirs's was like a brother and sister relationship. Latha felt further worst about her narrow mindedness. She continued to suffer in her mind. It was like hot ghee that you cannot swallow and cannot spit out also. As a result of this, her unhappiness continued and increased. This made Niranjan to bring her to me.

She felt very relieved when I said that I understood her feelings. She was happy that I didn't label her as narrow minded. We can recall that even her mother had advised her not to be narrow minded. She said that she was ashamed even to bring it up with her very good husband. I asked Latha whether she really felt that she was narrow minded contrary to whatever others said. She said that she didn't know. I told her that she was not at all narrow minded and anybody would have reacted in the same way.

In the next visit I explained to her that there were society norms in opposite sex relationships immaterial of the age. We are very close with our natural sisters. Why we do not feel same way with a different girl of same age? The difference in our reaction is a result of our upbringing in the society. We incorporate certain behaviors from observing others in the society. Our reactions are automatically carried out without our knowledge. I asked Latha if she had seen such a close relationship between an elderly man and a younger girl, who are not biologically related. She had never seen a such thing. It was unusual and unnatural. I found out Latha's relationship with her husband was excellent and she was comfortable to talk anything to him except this. I ascertained from her that she was not afraid of any repercussions if she talked to him. In psychotherapy we have to ascertain strengths and weaknesses in the marriage, before bringing it up with the spouse. If we do not ascertain it may cause an irreparable damage to their relationship. I encouraged her to talk to her husband in my presence and I would help her in that.

I called the husband inside and told him that we knew the problem and it required his participation and it required psychotherapy. He said that they didn't have much time as they were to leave India on an assignment abroad in 3 days. Both requested me to help them in that short time. At that time, I felt they were ready to handle it right away. They requested me to begin the treatment right away. I agreed to extend the session.

Niranjan promised that he will do whatever he can to make Latha happy and he will not take reprisal against her and he would take it with grace. I asked Latha to reveal the problem. Initially Niranjan felt bad about her narrow mindedness. I asked him how it could be narrow mindedness. He responded by saying what else it could it be, after all it was a pure brother and sister relationship. I asked him to imagine a situation where Latha was in such a pure relationship with a similarly aged boy. He was speechless. I insisted him to say whether it was alright with him. Finally he said that he wouldn't tolerate it. When it was not alright for him how it could be alright for her. I also told him that there were society norms, which we had to follow. All these society norms are to be followed in the interest of everybody in the society. He should also think of Meena's future also, if the matter spreads, she might have difficulty in her marriage prospects in future.

Niranjan seemed to understand. He felt sorry for his narrow mindedness. Now the narrow mindedness turned around the table to Niranjan himself. Niranjan felt ashamed of his narrow mindedness. I said that it was not narrow minded at all, but only society norms should be practiced with good intention or else it might have repercussions on others in the society. He agreed to discontinue his relationship with that girl and reiterated that his marriage harmony was more important. I was able to solve their problem in one extended session. This is the shortest successful psychotherapy session in my practice of over 4 decades. I felt quite happy with the outcome. They parted thanking me. I was surprised to see Latha in my clinic again after 5 months. They had returned from abroad and she said that she was passing by my clinic and thought of visiting me. She expressed that she was never so much happy as this in her life. She had come to thank me once again.

Psychodynamics

Let us try to understand their problems psychodynamically. In a happy marriage there was unhappiness. There was nothing to pinpoint the problem and even Latha was not aware of it properly. She was uncomfortable about the relationship of her husband with Meena. She felt narrow minded about their relationship and felt guilty for entertaining such thoughts. Latha's mother scolded her for her narrow mindedness and Latha's feeling of narrow mindedness increased. With all these Latha was not able to come to terms with her feelings. The question here is did she doubt her husband? I emphatically say "no" for this.

What she doubted was not her husband but his instincts. All of us have sexual instincts. These are biological. As stated in earlier chapters instincts are ID's nature and are primitive and has no value system. With the evolution of the society certain norms were practiced for the betterment of the society. The evolution of the society framed certain rules, which later followed blindly from generation to generation. The result was the formation of family, a unit of the society. Sex was considered taboo with the members of the family other than wife. For the primitive sexual instincts, society norms were the barriers. We can recall about Freud's superego here. When we are sleeping our ego also rests and we are afraid something unnatural may happen with the member of opposite sex, even with a blood relative. This is the exact reason why we don't allow opposite sex siblings to sleep in the same bed. The society doesn't encourage very much physical proximity between opposite sex siblings for the fear something unnatural may happen in a bad moment. Latha was afraid of Niranjan's instincts and not Niranjan. Her conflict between instincts and moral values of superego was not resolved and led to the problems.

Psychotherapy

The very first thing to be dealt was to focus on her inhibition and then she expressed her what was called by her as narrow mindedness.

She expressed this to her mother and was told that she was narrow mindedness and not trusting her husband. She felt miserable, because no one understood her feelings. She was made aware that it was not narrow mindedness of her at all and in fact it was a society norm. With this she could express her feelings freely. She had a good relationship with her husband and hence I decided to have a joint session to solve the problem. Latha had same typical feeling in our society not to disrespect the husband, even disagreeing on a relevant point is also considered by many as disrespecting. This had to be dealt with her. Her inhibitions had to be dealt with, for her to speak freely with her husband. When once the conflict became conscious the resultant anxiety disappeared. The resolution of the conflict brought about certain revelations and appropriate adjustments between Latha and her husband.

Being Poisoned

Raghu was a 30years old male. He was an accountant in a bank. All relatives were fond of him. He had a good income. He was considered as a good worker in the bank. He was recommended for promotion in the bank. Besides good work and well-paying job he was handsome also. He had fair colored skin with five and a half feet height and 145 pounds weight. Relatives were even telling their children to emulate him. There were matrimonial enquiries from girl's parents.

No human being is perfect. Everybody has some or the other deficiency. Raghu was unhappy and anxious for 6 months. His concentration decreased. His work efficiency reduced. He lost interest in everything in life. He had giddiness intermittently. He didn't improve with treatment from his family doctor. His problems got worsened. One of his friends suggested him to see a physician. The physician said that he had no physical problem and prescribed him some tonic for strength. When that didn't help he went to another two doctors and again didn't help. Someone suggested him to go to an ENT surgeon because he had giddiness. The ENT specialist said that he had no ENT problem. His problem continued to get worsened. If he read something it would keep ruminating in his mind. The sleep problem began. He began having bad dreams. Sometimes these bad dreams woke him up and could not fall asleep again. Unable to bear this he was applying leave from work. Because he was a good worker the bank manager initially was keeping quiet, but later the bank manager gave him warnings. Still later the manager told him that he had to take a tough action on him. His colleagues requested the manager to be considerate because Raghu had some troubles. The bank manager couldn't understand Raghu's problems as all doctors had declared that Raghu had no troubles. Finally the manager gave him one month leave and to return after getting well.

Raghu lost control over his mind and began day dreaming. In the night he was unable to sleep, and his restlessness started disturbing others. One night he began shouting. The other members woke up and were scared. The parents informed his elder sister and brother in law and requested them to come immediately. They had to come from another town, and they came the following morning. All the family members decided to take him for a vacation to a big city. Their contention was that Raghu needed rest and he would be alright. It didn't work and they consulted some doctors there also. Raghu began to laugh inappropriately. He would open the door and tried to go out at night. His sister and brother in law had to be awake the whole night in order to guard him. Sometimes he would shout and there were complaints from others. He began saying that he heard some body's voice when no one was in the vicinity. Even for a small sound Raghu was getting scared. If someone passed near, he would say they had come to kill him. He began claiming someone had put some poison in him and trying to kill him. The brother in law brought a person to remove poison from his body. That person gave something and made Raghu Vomit and said that he would be alright as poison was removed from the body. The problem continued and he kept saying that he was poisoned. The person who removes the poison was brought again and Raghu was made to vomit with no relief. Finally, they brought him to me on the advice of someone.

Raghu's brother in law was scared to bring him to my clinic because he was under the impression that my patients would be behaving very strange and weird like they show in movies. He thought that nobody who came to me would be acting normal.

Ours is a poly clinic and we have a common waiting hall for all the patients. Raghu's brother in law was surprised that he did not find any difference between my patients and other doctor's patients in the waiting hall. He later expressed to me that he felt bad at his ignorance. This is not uncommon because of social stigma and ignorance. He explained in detail Raghu's problem. While he was describing Raghu was preoccupied and looked as though it didn't belong to him. He was looking somewhere all the time. When I asked something, he responded by saying "what did you say?" He denied that his mind was brooding with something. He claimed that he was poisoned. He replied it was through the food about six months back. I asked him who he thought had poisoned him and his response was that it was someone who hated him. He didn't know who it was. I tried to find out how he came to that conclusion and his response was he was certain because he was experiencing all those symptoms. He had not found any change in the taste of food and there was no bad smell also. On examination he had no physical problem and had no effects of any poison. I wanted to admit him into the nursing home, but his brother in law requested me to treat him as an outpatient as they had incurred a lot of expenditure on him.

In the first two days I gave him antipsychotic medicines. We have to begin on a small dose and increase it as necessary till he became alright. The right dose necessary depended on many factors like body constitution, weight, tolerability, severity of illness, etc. In the first two days there was no remarkable improvement in Raghu's illness. His brother in law got worried and I had to educate him that medicines need time to be effective and also, he was on starter doses yet. I had to keep on increasing his medicines daily and on fourth day there was some improvement. He was more relaxed and slept for a few hours. On fifth day he was more cheerful. The voices and restlessness had not gone completely. When I asked him about being poisoned he said "may be. I may have been poisoned". I kept increasing his medicines as he was not alright yet.

Everybody's constitution is different. We cannot decide how much food one will eat by looking at a person. One may be hefty and eat less. Another person may be lean and may eat more. In the same way we cannot decide on the dose of medicine on seeing a person. Some people improve with small doses of medicine and another may need a lot more. Raghu gradually became alright. He was cheerful, sleep and appetite improved. When asked about his feeling of being poisoned he would say" I am not sure. It may be something else also". A week later he laughed and couldn't believe that he had said he was poisoned before.

Mere pharmacotherapy was not enough and in the hospital I treated him with some psychotherapy also. The first thing was educating him about poisons. Most of the poisons have a very bad smell and very bitter taste and it is very difficult to get a person to swallow that without his knowledge. Most of the poisons are very fast acting and Raghu's problem began six months before and in no way it was possible for that poison to remain in the body for that long. If he was really poisoned, he should have died a long ago. There was a question whether there were medicines that could cause mental disturbance. There are such medicines, but their actions are temporary. The action may wear off in about half hour to four hours. There are no such medicines that can cause a permanent mental disturbance. After he was convinced that being poisoned a remote possibility, he began saying that he might be killed in some other manner. So many people had been killed in six months and why it didn't happen to him? He had no answer. Even people with very high security had been killed and was it difficult to kill Raghu? I also told him that nobody tried to kill him in six months and yet he didn't leave his feeling of being killed. These revelations influenced Raghu.

Raghu became quite normal. I advised him to see me once a month for follow up. He began working as usual. I apprised him of the importance of taking medicines properly. His illness is Schizophrenia. In this illness regularly taking medicines is very important, because pharmacotherapy is most important in this illness. The recent studies indicate in Schizophrenia there is a biochemical imbalance with excessive production of serotonin (5 hydroxy tryptophan). Excessive serotonin is known to cause severe mental disturbance. In schizophrenia psychotherapy has a minimal role and pharmacotherapy is the main treatment. A schizophrenic has a lot of denial. He denies of having an illness and refuses to take medicines. Invariably they will have a poor follow up in the treatment. This poses a big difficulty for the family and doctors. The minimal role of psychotherapy can be of some use in a few patients. I have a few patients refusing to take medicines. At such times I have asked the family to call me and put me in contact with the patient over the phone. I advise the patient again the importance of taking the medicines and he follows. This may not work with all. This is called psychotherapeutic relationship between the psychiatrist and the patient. Raghu's family kept track of his medicine intake. Often the schizophrenic patient refuses to cooperate with the family for taking the medicines. Sometimes patient puts medicines in his mouth and spit them outside. The treatment of schizophrenia is a very long one. If he takes the medicine properly he can lead an almost normal life. Compliance with treatment is the most difficult problem in this illness, because of noncompliance repeated flare up in illness may happen. Many schizophrenics may require a lifelong maintenance dose of medicine. Raghu came for follow up for 4 months and he was alright. He didn't follow up further and hopefully he is alright.

Bad Omen

Somu aged 27 years complained of severe palpitation and chest pain for 2 years and it had worsened for 3 months. Nowadays it was unbearable. It was so severe, at times he felt as though his chest cage might break and he was afraid that he might die. Sometimes he even preferred death than bearing this suffering. He had consulted many general practitioners, physicians and even cardiologists. One cardiologist suggested him to see me. He and the whole family were disturbed about his illness. Their contention was that he had real pain and why he should be lying. It was not psychological(their word here was mad) according to them. All in the family concluded that all tests were normal and several doctors examinations did not find any physical illness, yet they were not ready to accept it could be psychological. They thought something was missed by all doctors. The family took him to astrologers and Curse removers with no avail. They took him to well-known cardiologists in other states. Meanwhile, they visited many temples and sacred worshipping places as per the advice of spiritual peoples and elders, but his suffering continued. Running out of all choices and in desperation they brought him to me with a thick file of medical records. The family felt it was not psychological as he had real pain. Somu was a young well-built unmarried man. He seemed to be dull and talked slowly. He said that he had lost interest in life. He preferred death instead of bearing this agony. He was shabbily dressed and engrossed. He was of average intelligence. He was very anxious. There was no psychosis. His higher mental functions like orientation, memory, judgment, etc were normal. I made a diagnosis of Depression with anxiety and psychosomatic symptoms. I put him on some antidepressant and antianxiety agents. I advised him to see me for once a week session for the next few weeks.

In the next session, Initially I had to reassure him that he had no physical problem and it was psychological. He was afraid that I had declared him as mad. This is a very common reaction amongst people. I had to explain to him that mental illness didn't mean madness. The science had advanced tremendously. There were so many psychological problems other than madness or insanity as he thought. I assured him that his was definitely not madness. He seemed to become more comfortable with me. He had some questions regarding the treatment

I explained to him that he had problem for 2 years and it was severe for 3 months and it could not be solved in one or two visits. The medicines were given for some relief for the present. Medicines are only temporary and symptomatic relief. He was advised psychotherapy for lasting relief (It is popularly known as Talk therapy and also as counseling in the society). He admitted that he becomes tense and depressed. He was advised to see me once a week therapy sessions for a few weeks. Then I called his relatives inside. I had to explain once again to thwart their ignorance about mental illness. It is not uncommon initially we may have to spend a lot of time with relatives also. It is very exhaustive and two such families a day will be brain storming for a psychiatrist. I was able to convince them to bring him back to subsequent therapy sessions.

In the next few sessions, Somu was more comfortable and more expressive. I encouraged him to express all of his mental agony. He had lost his father 4 yrs before. He was living with mother, 3 brothers and 2 sisters. He expressed theirs was an affectionate family. He couldn't finish high school. He had a small business for 3 years of buying and selling gold. He wanted to go to a government job, but not able to get any for his qualification. His business had improved and able to earn enough to pay rent and contribute some for the family maintenance. Thematic apperception test revealed that he was less bold and less expressive of anger. He expressed anxiety, mind disturbed, fear, unhappiness, poor sleep and mind not under control. All these are symptoms of psychological problem, specifically Depression.

In psychotherapy, psychiatrist has to keep observing all the thoughts of the patient. Sometimes a matter is expressed in a seemingly unrelated manner. If we put all of them together and observe it might give some clue. In one session casually talking he said that there were a lot of crows in front of his shop. He was afraid the crow might come inside, and it may result in loss of his business. The entrance of a crow inside is considered as a bad omen. Lately his business had improved. There were about 30 such shops in the area and still his business had improved well. He was afraid that he might lose his business, if crows enter his shop.

His was a small shop of 6 ft x 5 ft. He was alone in the shop and there was not enough room to have a helper also. His shop was opened from 9.30 AM to 9 PM. His residence was 7 kilometers away and couldn't go home for lunch. In a day he would get about 20 customers. He had 5 customers from 9.30 am to 6.00 pm. There were about 15 customers from 6 PM to 9 PM. He had a lot of time in between and felt bored. He expressed it was very frustrating. He couldn't reduce the hours also as It was a very competitive business and couldn't afford even a loss of a couple of customers. He had no habit of reading books or magazines for spending free time at work. At this stage his fear of crows entering inside the shop began. He was afraid it might hurt his business. He also expressed that he had dreams of crows entering his shop. The question that I had in my mind was that he had this business for 3 years and the crows were there always, then why he had fears for 3 months only. If it is purely fear of bad omen it should have been there from the beginning itself. This meant there was something more to it than just fear of bad omen. Besides this the crows had not really entered his premises. I tried to find out if he believed in bad omen always. He said that he never really believed it before, but for 3 months he believed it. He reported that he heard from a known person that a crow had come inside his premises and nothing had happened to his business or family. With this piece of information, he also felt nothing might happen to him also.

In the next session I raised the issue that he was afraid of bad omen in one part of the mind and a feeling of nothing might happen in another part of the mind. He agreed readily. At this stage I raised a question if there could be any other reason for this. In return he asked me what the reason could be. I told him at that stage both of us were not aware of the reason and both of us should work towards it. He was prepared to do anything to solve his problem. I was happy with his determination to solve his problem; this indicated a strong motivation in him to seek solution to his problem. I wanted to know what he was afraid might happen if a crow came inside. He expressed that he was afraid it might result in loss of his business. He denied any other harm that could happen. That means it was a selective fear. So many other things could also happen, but why he had only this fear was a big question. Whenever there is a conflict our unconscious mind selects a fear which would serve a hidden purpose. At this stage I had some idea about his problem. Our unconscious wishes might reflect as fears (Sigmund Freud). This is difficult to digest, isn't it? The question was why his unconscious mind might be wishing for the loss of his business and his conscious mind didn't want his business to be spoiled. This was also true. At this stage we needed to explore further why the part of his mind had some negative feelings about his business. What he was aware at that stage was fear of loss of his business

Further sessions threw some light. He began cursing himself for not pursuing his education and if he had pursued education he would have been in a better position in life. He felt sorry that he was stuck in this business, but he had no choice. I told him that there was no point in repenting about the past and to think of only what he could do at the present. Generally, people ponder too much about their inactions of the past. He had a lot of free time in the shop and most of the time he was spending watching people walking outside. Some time he had thought of closing his business and find a job, even if it fetched less income. The family said how he could close a good income business. It was also question of survival. The family would tell him he was not in his good senses to close a good income business. They even cautioned him that the family might have to go hungry if he closed the business. In a way Somu also agreed internally. He sought the opinion about his problem with some of the elders in his extended family. He presented them his vacillation about his business. The elders also advised him not to close the business because there was no other alternative. This kept on going with many of his people. He couldn't decide and this conflict continued. Suddenly one day it dawned in his mind if a crow came inside his shop. At this stage his symptoms began, and he began having severe palpitations and fear that his chest may break also.

At this stage we should watch his flow of thoughts. At first, he had a conflict whether to continue his business or close it. He couldn't come to any decision. At this time, he developed fear of crow entering the shop. His unconscious mind grabbed the idea of fear of crow and conscious mind didn't want to for realistic reasons. If the crow could make the decision for him, it spared him from blaming himself. He could blame the bad omen. Human being doesn't want to blame himself. People commonly would like to blame fate, bad luck and bad omen for their problems. It is unacceptable to blame himself for any problem. We call this as displacement (The real blame is displaced on to the bad omen), which is one of the Ego mechanisms to deal with the stress. Awareness of this had significant effect.

In the next visit Somu was quite cheerful. He reported that his fear of crow was gone. He agreed that he had a conflict about his business. It was necessary for survival, but extremely boring. He thought over certain things. He wanted to take up a job, but couldn't get any job that would pay at least to match his present income. He told that he decided to stick to the business. He mentioned that there is no scope for improving his business. I raised a point whether he could find a way to occupy himself in the free time in business. He could develop a hobby. I saw him after a month, and he was completely alright. He reported he had decided to read some magazines and installed a television to ward off his boredom.

Psychodynamics

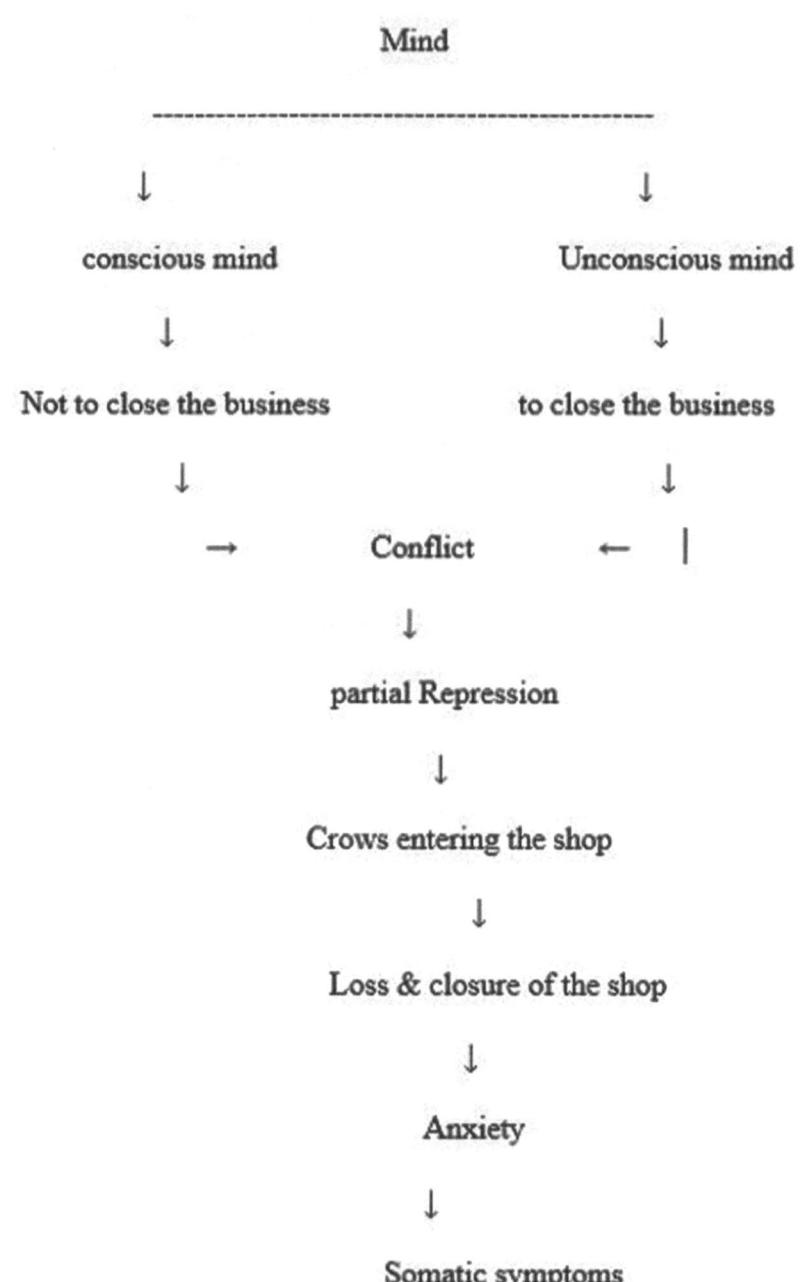

His conscious mind vacillated between not closing and closing the business. For realistic factors he decided partially to continue the business. It was not acceptable to another part of the mind. This part of the mind repressed the idea and went into the unconscious mind. It began giving trouble in a hidden manner. This part of the mind grabbed the idea of crows entering and thus bad omen. In this way he could blame the bad omen and spare himself from blaming. The conflict was created between the conscious and unconscious minds. The unconscious mind did not reconcile to continue the business. The conflict led to anxiety and somatic symptoms.

Psychotherapy

The first step in all psychotherapies is ventilation. The patient was allowed to talk about his illness. Ventilation eases the mind to some extent. This is called as Catharsis. Somu expressed about his agony from his symptoms like anxiety, palpitation and chest pain. After that I raised a question as to what he thought was responsible for his problem. Of course, his answer was negative. The reason why I asked the question was to make his mind inquisitive about his illness.

Somu was educated as to the conscious and unconscious parts of the mind. It was brought to his awareness the relationship between the mind and body. Since he was cleared of any physical illness the alternative left was mind. He was aware of two opposite views on his business in the conscious mind. As one part of the conscious mind decided to stick with his business, the other part of the conscious mind was adamant. This part of the mind went into the unconscious part by a mechanism of repression. Somu's mind was trying to get unconsciously what it could not get consciously.

The conflict began between conscious and unconscious minds. The unconscious mind grabbed on the idea of crows and bad omen. The mind is selfish and illogical to achieve its goals. Here the unconscious mind selfishly wanted to close the business and seek a job. Illogically it grabbed the idea of bad omen at this time, even though the crows were present from the beginning of his business. The crows didn't enter the premises at all. This weakened the intensity of his unconscious mind and yet it didn't reconcile. The conflict continued. An impossible situation resulted. He had anxiety, palpitation and chest pain.

Somu became aware of this unconscious mind in therapy. The two parts of the mind acting against each other was his problem. This awareness resulted in harmony between the two parts of the mind. He finally decided once again to stick to his business. He took measures to deal with his free time in his business.

Pinching Disease

There is stigma and ignorance on mental illness. Many people think it is a curse of god, devil's possession, madness, poisoning and it is an act of unnatural spirit. People are subjected to treatment from spiritual persons, charlatans, poison removers etc. They are brought to a psychiatrist after running out of all choices. Those who had close experience of psychiatric treatment have a much different approach. It will have a better impact on a prospective patient when it comes from another cured patient.

One gentleman brought a lady along with her son and daughter to me. He said that I had treated his daughter and she was fine. They were his relatives and knew the plight of their problem. He introduced them to me and went out. The patient, Saroja, a 55 years old female was murmuring herself, which was not understandable. She was in her own world. She was not able to express properly. She would ask a question and kept asking the same again and again even when I answered it. She had a problem of pinching people. If anybody didn't go along with her she would pinch them. She would pinch people in bus, neighbors, etc. Because of this problem some family member had to be with her always. Her pinch was never serious enough to cause any wound, but was painful.

Saroja claimed her food was poisoned and would pinch a lot to the person who served food. She would shout loud and even the neighbors were concerned as to what was happening. Her children and husband failed to convince her against pinching. Out of frustration her husband hit her mildly and she started saying "see, he is trying to kill me'. It was getting worse as the days passed. She was pinching and shouting for trivial reasons. Some time when she was eating she would count one, two, and three like that and stop eating. She was always counting less than ten. She had sleep difficulty also. Sometimes she would get up at 2 or 3 am chanting something loudly and worshipping god. This would disturb the sleep of others. Because of this behavior family thought it was some god's curse and sought treatment from spiritual healers. The family took her to temples, church, mosque, etc with no improvement.

Often saroja scolded others as devil. The family took treatment from people who claimed to take out devil from the person supposed to be possessed by devil. It was thought it could be the act of bad spirit and treatment from those healers had no effect. I can go on all other types of treatment Saroja was subjected to. It would be a separate book by itself. She was admitted to a mental hospital for one month. The medicines were not helpful and the psychiatrist advised her shock treatment (electroconvulsive therapy). The family was against it and got her discharged.

Saroja was a lean built lady with 5 feet height and about 100 pounds weight. She had grey hairs and bad teeth. I found out she had a heart problem. She looked older than her age. As usual I wanted to see her privately. The family was worried she might pinch me. I had handled a lot of violent patients in my practice. I told them that I would manage and to stay outside for a while. Even as they were going out Saroja shouted at them to come back. She attained menopause 3 years ago. She was treated by a cardiologist about one year ago. Her problem began three years ago. She never had any emotional problems before three years. Her adjustment in the family was excellent before three years. She was irrelevant and psychotic. Her problem is called as involutional psychosis. Her illness was severe, but I hesitated from giving shock treatment because of her heart problem. The treatment risk for life is high in such cases. I prescribed antipsychotic medicines and sent her home. She was brought back within no time saying she was unmanageable. They requested me to admit her. I admitted her in a nursing home and began treating with medicines. She developed some side effects and I had to start her on another medicine. Her condition was not brought under control and other patients in the nursing home began complaining about her pinching.

The family was getting fed up and her problem was getting worse. The only alternative left was shock treatment. I was also worried about the risk involved. I had a meeting with all family members to discuss about shock treatment and risks involved in particular with her. The family was ready this time. I had to explain the risk of life involved. They were ready out of sheer frustration. I ordered for tests like brain scan, chest x ray, blood and urine examinations. All were negative. I had a discussion with anesthetist and cardiologist. They gave a green signal for the shock treatment. After all these were done the family had second thoughts and decided against shock treatment and had her discharged. After a couple of days they brought her back and agreed for shock treatment. They were unable to manage her.

This treatment had to be given in a full-fledged hospital facility to handle any eventuality. I gave first treatment in the presence of anesthetist and cardiologist. It was successful. I had to give four more treatments at intervals. Her pinching behavior reduced.. She became more relevant and was able to understand when she was told something. She was not completely alright. Once there was a relapse. Two more shock treatments were given and she became alright. She was discharged. The family took her to different places without any problem. The family couldn't believe the change in her. When the family brought her for follow up they said that they never had a peaceful meal like this in last three years.

Involutional psychosis affects at menopausal and later ages. The woman's body goes through a disturbance in the body. There is a lot of hormonal and biochemical changes during menopause. It is a very stressful time for a woman's body. Women in menopause have a lot of psychological and physical problems. Some professionals feel it is a variant of schizophrenia, but occurring in a later age. I treated Saroja about 35 years ago. Those days psychopharmacology was not so much advanced. We didn't have so many wide variety and good medicines as of now. Less numbers of medicines were available and whatever medicines available were in minimum doses. One medicine was available in 25 mg tablets only. Sometimes we had to give 200 mg four times a day. That meant I had to give 8 tablets four times day. Imagine the plight of a patient if a doctor prescribed 8 tablets four times a day? Anybody would get frightened, because of this shock treatment was necessary in those days. Today's patient has a better choice of medicines. The prognosis is very good nowadays. If I were to treat her today I would confidently say I would manage with medicines only. I have not given any shock treatment in the last two decades of my practice.

Mind Reading

Rojan, a 30 years old man came with his father. His father was a pharmacist and he knew me. Rojan lived with his parents. He had studied Bachelor of business management (BBM) and was unemployed. His mother was a home maker. He had no siblings. He had thyroid deficiency and diabetes. He was under treatment for them. He chewed tobacco 4 times and smoked 2 cigarettes per day.

Father said Rojan claimed that people cursed him. He had been under the treatment of another psychiatrist for 6 years. Six years earlier he heard voices, cut the sarees and broke vessels. He had improved, but not completely alright. He continued to say people cursed him; they read his mind and had poor sleep. Rojan claimed that somebody had implanted something in the house. They changed the house, but the troubles continued.

Rojan spoke well in the absence of his father. He said people read his mind. He was scared. People knew whatever he had thought. He was free of the voices now. He was calm and could express well. He was very disturbed about people reading his mind. His higher mental functions were alright. I viewed his earlier treatment records. I agreed with previous psychiatrist's diagnosis of schizophrenia. The previous psychiatrist had given proper medications for the problem. What more I could do? I decided not to change his medications and try to deal with him about his symptoms.

In the next two sessions I Just allowed him to talk. He went on describing about others reading his mind. While walking if a lady passed by his side from the opposite side he had to look at her, he thought other people felt he was looking sexually at that lady. He asked how he could go without seeing her. He had looked at her casually just like looking at others. He said others were mistaking him. He said looking at women in a sexual manner was very wrong. He said people cursed him thinking he was ogling at women. He said several people had thought he was staring at women.

At the end of second session he asked me what I felt about people reading his mind. I asked him how convinced he was in this belief of others reading his mind. He said he was 100% sure. If he was so sure, why he asked me for my opinion? This showed there was some element of doubt in him. He agreed. I told him it was impossible for any person to read another person's mind. He wanted to test it between ourselves first. He kept quiet and thought of something without saying anything. He asked me what he had thought. I told him I didn't know what he had thought. Then he wanted to test if he could read my mind. He asked me to think of something and I did. I asked him if he could read what I was thinking. He said he could not read my mind.

He continued saying people were reading his mind. I told him all people were created by nature in a similar way and no one could read other's minds. His mind was not a computer screen where anyone could read. He was concerned people would know his thoughts; it meant he was scared of people coming to know his thoughts. The question what was he hiding or ashamed of ? He said people thought he looked at women in a sexual manner. Of all the things why he was thinking of this? It meant he was trying to communicate something about women.

We spent sometimes talking about general things about women. After a long time he said it was bad to even think of women. He said sexual matters should be in the framework of marriage only. Then slowly he revealed he gets the names of some women, but never names of men. After a long time, he said that he got dreams of women. He hated it. These bad dreams were disturbing him and woke him up. At this stage it was clear about his fear of people coming to know his thoughts. He admitted of having sexual thoughts on women. He considered himself as a very bad person.

I had to educate him that everyone got sexual thoughts and attractions as it was a biological instinct. No one could avoid it. He quoted some books and vedantas (spiritual sayings), which depicted even to have sexual thoughts were wrong. A lot of people argue they never get such thoughts. They are not true to themselves and they draw innocent people like Rojan into a confused path.

My counseling influenced Rojan gradually. His sleep improved. He didn't block his thoughts. Human mind is strange. If you allow your thoughts freely after some time they will not be enticing any more. What is prohibited is more enticing. Rojan's trouble was his instinctual mind (ID) got sexual thoughts and his rigid moral mind (Superego) was trying to ban it from conscious mind. The adult mind (EGO) was not able to resolve it. Rojan became peaceful in his mind and I terminated psychotherapy, but continued to see him for psychopharmacotherapy once a month in the beginning and now once in three months.

What I have narrated it looks so simple. To convince even a neurotic individual is very difficult. To convince a schizophrenic is extremely difficult. Their defense mechanisms of denial and projection make it very difficult to convince. It took me 22 psychotherapy sessions to convince Rojan for above matter. The readers can imagine how difficult it was. When it is reported in a summary it looks so simple. It requires a lot of time and patience to explore and convince a patient. I can't describe this frustration in words. In schizophrenia the prime and most important treatment is medications. Psychotherapy can play an important secondary role in some patients like Rojan

Breathlessness and Palpitation

It was a Saturday, last day of the week. Usually Saturdays are busy. On that Saturday my scheduled appointments were medium. I was happy I could go early home and spend more time with my family. When I was thinking like that my receptionist told me that I had a call from Dr Thomas. I answered the phone call. Dr Thomas said that there was a person from Fiji and requested me to see him that day itself. He was admitted in a nursing home where I was a consultant. The patient had come here for treatment and had to go back soon.

I went to the nursing home after my clinic. Dr Thomas introduced me to the patient. His name was Fr. John. He was a priest. For one-year Fr. John had breathlessness and palpitation and it had worsened in the last one month. Dr Thomas had run all tests and a physical examination didn't reveal any physical illness. I and Dr Thomas had a discussion and decided Fr. John required psychiatric intervention.

Fr John was about 5 feet height with 125 pounds weight. He greeted me with a sweaty hand. He talked with a very low voice and was stammering at times. His hands were shaking, and he looked very anxious. He seemed to be afraid of something. I asked him to be seated on a chair and I sat on another chair. His problems began with sleep difficulty about a year ago. If he slept well one day he had difficulty in sleep on the next day. It had been getting worse lately and almost every day he had sleep difficulty. He would wake up in the morning feeling as if he had not slept at all that night. A month after the sleep problem began; he woke up one night with catching of breath and palpitation. Lately it had become an everyday affair. He would have breathing difficulty with pulling sensation of the muscles. He was profusely sweating. He was getting fear he might die. The palpitation was so severe he felt it was heart attack. He was seen by doctors in Fiji and was told it was just a weakness. He was prescribed some tonics. Fr John's problem kept increasing and was not bearable.

Fr john was born in kerala. His parents were Christians and wanted him to be a big priest and helpful to others. Being an obedient person, Fr John had fulfilled the parents dream. His parents expired. He didn't have any siblings. He got involved more in serving people. Recognizing his service, the higher order in the church sent him to Fiji about 5 years ago. He became very popular in Fiji because of selfless service. He came here for learning more about Christianity. He was to return to Fiji in six days. He denied of any worries. He didn't remember the dreams that he had. I tried to find out if he had any reservations about going back to Fiji. But he was eager to go back.

On examination I didn't find any physical illness. He had no neurological illness also. He had physical symptoms and it could be due to either physical illness or it could be due to psychological problem. We had ruled out any physical illness. I was left with only possibility of psychological. Sleeplessness, anxiety and hands shaking pointed towards psychological problem, but he denied of any worries. How to get it out was a challenge. This is a problem each and every psychiatrist faces every day with most of his patients.

I administered TAT(thematic apperception) test on him. I showed a few pictures and asked him to tell all that came to his mind. In this test we ask the patient to build stories as he could imagine. The way he builds up stories it gives us some idea about his problems. I learnt there was some sexual issue in Fr John. The patient was not aware of it. As he had to go back in six days, I was trying to accelerate the therapy. I decided to subject him to narcoanalysis.

In this test a medicine called pentothal is injected to make his conscious mind sleep. Then the unconscious mind comes out without any inhibitions. It serves the same purpose as hypnosis. It is achieved by pharmacological means. It is a further development of hypnosis. It is more successful than hypnosis. Hypnosis requires full cooperation and concentration of the patient. He has to follow our instruction diligently. Narcoanalysis requires his physical submission and it is faster. If the patient has some physical problems like heart problem we have to be cautious, otherwise this is preferred nowadays. It is used in criminology a lot.

I subjected him to narcoanalysis on the next day, even though it was a Sunday. I had the responsibility for augmenting his therapy. He was talking to nuns (Christian ladies devoted to the religious cause) about 1.5 years ago. His talking with nuns had increased. Gradually it turned to flirting. He had some enjoyment in it. He was attracted to one. He had very strong moral values. He felt it was sinful even to think sexually and on the other hand he was attracted. He felt remorseful. I discharged him from the nursing home and asked him to see me in my clinic.

He was eager to know what he had said in narcoanalysis. I revealed it and he admitted it was true. He knew that he enjoyed flirting with one nun, but he never realized there was sexual inclination in it. He revealed that he had two times dreams of sexual involvement with that nun. When he had those dreams, he felt very bad for himself. He tried hard to control those feelings. Those feelings continued and kept increasing. As those feelings increased his breathlessness and palpitations increased. He felt very remorseful and hated himself. He expressed that he was a sinner and unfit to be a priest, even though he had never indulged in any sexual act.

Almost all religions preach one should be pure in mind also. One is not supposed to have any bad thoughts. Is it practical and possible? Priests are also human beings. They bequeath usual pleasures. Can they bequeath certain thoughts also? Isn't' it our expectation is too much on them? Our society's expectation on them is too much. If anybody says he thinks of only good thoughts and never had any bad thoughts, he is either lying or fooling himself unconsciously. Both common and uncommon men are not very different psychologically. Both have good and bad thoughts. The uncommon man doesn't succumb to those thoughts; whereas the common man succumbs to those thoughts. Our control on actions is indicative of our strong ego development. Fr John had a very strong ego development. Fr John agreed with all the above of our discussion. He felt being in such a sacred position he shouldn't have such thoughts. He was not ready to accept it. Is there anyone who can follow 100% of what religion says? For ex;- all religions say love everyone. It is good and there is no doubt. Is it possible to love a murderer? All religions are good but we have to be realistic also. Our staunch religious beliefs take us too far. Fr John was able to understand. I told him to discuss this with other priests if he still had doubts.

It was 4th visit and Fr John was happy and said that he was 75% better. He had talked to a priest and also a friend about this and they told him the same also. He was relieved. He had accepted that the thoughts and actions should not be seen in the same way. He accepted the controls should be on actions. He had another issue to discuss on that day. He was afraid that all thoughts would lead to actions. I said it was not true. We think a whole lot and only a very few result in actions. If all thoughts were resulting in actions this world would have been impossible to live. Our mind should be free to think even bad things also. Our controls should be on actions. If we do not accept bad thoughts and push them to unconscious mind they may find expression with more vigor.

On the 5th and the last day Fr. John came and thanked me. He had talked to a higher order priest. He said that Fr John had not committed any sin. This also satisfied him. He was free of breathlessness and palpitations. He was quite confident and there was liveliness on his face. Fr John was to go back to Fiji very next day. I wished happy journey and all the best in the future. I terminated the therapy. I received a Christmas greeting from him with a note he was alright.

Some questions may arise in readers. Was Fr John a lier? Why did he hide his attraction to nuns from me? In TAT there was some information about sexual problem and even then why he didn't disclose it? Fr John was definitely not a liar. What he would gain by lying?. If he wanted to hide he would have discontinued the therapy. Why he should go through all the tests and spend so much money for just lying?. His cooperation suggests that he genuinely wanted a cure. He was not aware of his flirting with nuns had an underlying sexual attraction in it. It was possible because of his high moral values conflicted with unconscious sexual instincts. What is not acceptable to the conscious mind is pushed into the unconscious mind by a defense mechanism called Repression. If the repression is full it may never come to the conscious mind at all. If repression is partial it threatens to become conscious at different times. This generates anxiety, which further leads to all the problems like that of Fr John. There was also denial (another defense mechanism) in Fr John. He denied having sexual feeling. Another defense mechanism he used was splitting. He considered his flirting with nuns was nothing but flirting and had no sexual feeling in it. He could not maintain the homeostasis of the mind that way as his repression was only partial and it kept threatening to become conscious. We call a lie when done consciously and it is deliberate. The person knows it is a lie, but doesn't admit outwardly. In Fr John it was not a lie as he didn't even know it.

Psychodynamics

Human being is an instinctual individual and sexual instinct is one of them (ID). Even god men like priests cannot escape sexual instincts. Human being is a society (superego) individual also. The moral values of the society often cause conflicts. When both ID and Superego become unyielding the conflict is created. The conflict leads to anxiety. The anxiety in turn often leads to somatic problems as in Fr. John. Here both ID and Superego were acting unconsciously causing conflict. Both of them became conscious. The Superego became less harsh and natural instinct was accepted.

Psychotherapy

Fr. John was in India for six months. He was attracted to nun in Fiji. He was away from her and why he had the fear? In fact, he didn't have the fear and it emerged again as the date of returning to Fiji was nearing. He was scared of facing the situation of facing the nun. Fr john realized in therapy the root cause of his problem. Secondly, he realized that priest was also a man like anybody else. Thirdly he realized thought of a bad thing was not same as doing it. Fourthly he realized all thoughts do not result in actions. Finally, he realized that our control should be on action and not on thoughts.

Body Odour

A 50 years old man introduced himself as a professor in a college. He introduced his son, Mohan. Mohan was suffering from a bad body odor. Mohan kept complaining to parents a bad body smell was emanating from him. He complained that people were holding their noses and made faces if he passed by them. He was taken to his family physician, who said there was no disease that accounted for his alleged bad body odor. The father thought it might be better to see a dermatologist because the odor was coming from a skin problem. The Dermatologist cleared him of all skin problems. Mohan's problem continued. The father took him to another dermatologist and he also said that he couldn't find any health issues that could be responsible for it. This dermatologist advised Mohan to take good bath with plenty of soap. Mohan was already doing it. The whole family was an educated family and they were quite clean and had good hygienic habits. The dermatologist had prescribed some medicines and ointment, which did not help. Finally, the Dermatologist suggested his father to take him to a psychiatrist. It is not at all uncommon for almost all our patients to have had all types of treatments before coming to a psychiatrist.

As usual I sent his father out and spoke to Mohan alone. He said bad odor was coming out of the whole body. The bad odor was coming out of hairs, skin, nose and all other parts of the body. I didn't sense any bad odor emanating from him. He said people couldn't stand him because of this odor. He told that people would hold their noses and move away from him. The bad odor came out of his even clothes, school bag and stockings. Every day he took good bath with plenty of soap and yet the odor continued. He wore clean clothes daily, in spite of this there was a bad odor. He felt his odor was so bad it would not go even after washing his clothes. I asked him how he knew that bad odor was emanating from him. He said wherever he went there was bad odor and hence it must be coming out of him only. For my question he couldn't describe what kind odor it was. At a later point he said it was like that of rotten food type of odor. Mohan said he had no worries. He loved his parents and they cared for him very much. His sleep, appetites were normal. He was of more than average intelligence. There was no psychosis. His higher mental functions were alright. He was a less talkative person. His outstretched hands were shaking. I did not notice any bad body odor emanating from him. I called his father back to my chamber. I explained to them that mind was very powerful and we had to explore further in psychotherapy. I prescribed an antianxiety medicine and asked him to see me next week.

In the next visit Mohan looked cheerful and his bad odor had disappeared. He was very happy that I had given the right medicine to him. I explained to him and his father the medicine given was for the mind and not for the bad body odor. That meant I was in right tract and proved that his problem was psychological. Both of them didn't want any treatment as his problem was solved. They wanted a cure and it was already there. I had given a prescription for one week.

Mohan was not brought to me for next two months. He was brought to me again saying in spite of taking those medicines his problem got worsened. He had been continuing those medicines for two months (I had prescribed for one week only) as per the parents own decision. It is not uncommon for the patients to keep on taking medicines without the knowledge of the doctor. I had a patient who saw me once only and kept taking the medicines for about 5 years as he was alright with them. He had to come finally because that medicine was no longer manufactured by the company. I tried to find out the circumstances in which Mohan was experiencing bad body odor. It was unsuccessful. I had to increase his medicines as his problem had gotten worsened.

Again, I didn't see him for the next three weeks even though I had advised him to be brought one week later. The increased doses of medicines had helped and they neglected. The parents continued to give the same higher dose of medicine on their own decision. Again, the symptoms worsened and this time the parents were scared as to what would happen if medicines were continued in higher and higher doses. Sometimes the body develops resistance to the medicine and higher doses might be needed. I explained to them what they were doing was wrong. If a problem was not solved in the initial stages, it might become chronic with a lot more complications. The medicines are only temporary and symptomatic treatment. The root cause of the problem should be explored for a permanent cure. This time they were ready to follow my advice. I explained Mohan about treatment of psychotherapy.

Mohan came after one week and this time he had stopped medicines to see if he was going to be alright. His problem got worse. I told both him and his father not to meddle with the treatment. This time both were ready. This kind of erratic follow up of treatment is common in our society. I explained the importance of telling each and everything that came to his mind. Mohan didn't know what to talk for a while. He thought that he should continuously talk. He felt his father was paying money for talking and by not talking he thought he was wasting father's money. Many people think this way. One should express in talking, but to talk just for the sake of talking is not right. One should talk in a relaxed manner and be natural in their actions and expressions.

In the next few therapy sessions I posed certain points for his consideration as below: -

1. His bad body odor was sensed by him only, but nobody else told him. Why others had not mentioned of any bad odor coming out of him?

2. If others closed their noses, did it mean it was because of his body odor? Was it possible it might be their habit and he might be mistaking it?

3. Our mind controls the body. It can make us see things which are not there. A person going out at middle of the night may see something white moving at a distance and when he goes near there is nothing. We call this as illusion. In the same way Mohan might be feeling the bad odor in the same way. His sensing the odor was true, but it might be an illusion?

4. This bad odor emanated from what part of the body?

5. If the bad odor continued what was he afraid might happen?

Mohan said that nobody had told that a bad body odor was emanating from him. He said that he was not imagining and not lying. I told him that he was not lying at all. Why should he lie? It might be an illusion also. He argued that people really were closing their noses when he is nearer to him. I raised a question how did he know it was because of his bad odor they were holding their nose? Only those people who were doing it knew why they were holding their noses. I told him that I had not felt any bad odor coming out of him. He confirmed that his parents also said the same. He had asked a couple of his close friends and they also told him they had not felt any bad odor from him.

Mohan continued to believe that he had a bad body odor. He argued that I was not feeling the bad odor because it was controlled by medicines. I had to explain the medicine that I gave was for his anxiety and not for bad body odor. There was no medicine for controlling bad odor. He seemed to be out of any more excuses and asked me what I thought. I told him that it was his imagination that he had bad body odor. He said that I had a point, but he said that he was not lying. I agreed he was not lying at all. I explained to him lying is a deliberate act in a fully conscious state of the mind. Mohan's problem was in unconscious mind. I had to educate him about the structure of the mind. He was not even aware of the presence of an unconscious mind. When it happens in unconscious mind it is not at all lying. He had to be educated as to the relationship between the mind and body. I explained to him how the unconscious mind influences our sensory organs like nose.

Earlier Mohan had said the bad odor was like that of some rotten food. What did it mean? If bad odor was like that of rotten food did it mean he was something bad like rotten food? In other words did it mean Mohan felt so bad about himself on something like the smell of rotten food? It was only my thought at that time. I did not tell him anything. We shouldn't tell anything unless we are sure. He couldn't say from what part it was emanating. He also didn't say what damage it could cause.

In the next two therapy sessions again, he talked about his bad odor. He was found to be uncomfortable. I thought he would say something on his uncomfortable ness. I also kept quiet to see what he would do. He became more uncomfortable. I felt he wanted to say something and was not able to say. I told him he should say everything on his mind. He said "doctor if I tell you I hope you will not feel bad about me". I assured him being a psychiatrist I would not formulate such opinions. In a shrill voice he said that he was masturbating and that was the cause for the bad odor. He talked as though he had committed some crime. I assured him there was no need to feel bad about revealing this. He felt relieved. He told me that I was like his father and if I didn't mistake he would like to tell something. I promised I would not mistake. He had been masturbating for one year. He had read that masturbation was wrong. He wanted to stop. Without his realization he would masturbate in his sleep and ejaculate. When he woke up he felt nauseated because of the bad smell of the ejaculated fluid. He felt that odor was similar to the bad body odor that was coming out of his body.

In the next therapy session I had to deal with his ignorance on masturbation. First of all I told him masturbation was not wrong and most of the boys indulge in masturbation. He was scared to ask his parents. He read it in a magazine that masturbation was bad and harmful. Kinsey's study reported 92% of the boys and 60% of the girls masturbated. He was surprised at this information. He wanted to confirm again with me that masturbation was not harmful. I told him again it was not harmful at all and his source of information was wrong. He revealed that he had read it in some magazine. One should not read unauthentic magazines. At first Mohan didn't believe what I said. He thought that I was telling to please him. I told him that he could verify it from authentic sources like Indian psychiatric society. This made him believe what I said was correct. Some of these magazines report wrong things to propagate their circulation. Our society also behaves as if sexual matter is taboo and acts as if it should not be even talked about. The parents and in schools there is no mention of normal and appropriate sexual information. The result is that children fall prey to such bad magazines. The children are inquisitive and find information from wrong sources if we don't provide proper information.

Mohan talked about the odor of the ejaculation fluid (semen). Semen has its own smell. Mohan felt it had a bad smell because he thought masturbation was wrong and hence semen coming out of it must also be wrong. He was known as Mr. clean because he wouldn't even look at any girl. He admitted that he was staring at girls without the knowledge of others. He was upset about staring at girls and masturbation made him feel further bad. Mohan argued sexual interest before marriage was wrong. I asked him to tell what was right. He said he didn't know. How can a person say it is wrong when he doesn't know what is right? He slowly realized his ignorance. His next question was why semen should have that smell. It is body's creation and we had to accept it and we cannot change it. He accepted the natural odor of semen and stopped feeling it was a bad smell. How can the odor of semen come out of skin, etc? It was only his assumption. He believed masturbation and discharge of semen caused destruction of the body and a destroyed body emanating a body odor. That bad body odor was like that of semen. Mohan was of the opinion anything about sex was wrong. He felt that discharge of semen out of sexual stimulation was wrong. He had felt his masturbation had destroyed his body and hence bad odor was coming out of destroyed parts of the body. His complaints of bad body odor stopped. I terminated the therapy.

When I put it in summary about him it looks so simple. Why Mohan didn't tell his parents? How many parents are ready to discuss sexual matters with their children? Most of the parents are not comfortable to talk such things to the children as sexual matters are taboo. We do not reveal even normal sexual matters to children. Age appropriate knowledge can prevent a lot of problems.

Psychodynamics

Mohan consulted me for bad body odor problem. It was learnt later that it was related to his masturbation and discharge of semen. Normal sexual fantasies and acts like masturbation are age appropriate. He believed all sexual matters were taboo because they were bad. The natural sexual instinct (ID) could not be controlled by moral values (Superego). The result was conflict between ID and Superego. His Ego was not able to resolve the conflict because both parts of the minds were unyielding. The resulting anxiety made him disturbed and found expression in feeling that the body was destroyed. A spoiled body (like stale food) caused bad odor according to him. His ID was acting unconsciously, and Superego was acting consciously. Educating him about the normal and age appropriate sexual instincts weakened both ID and Superego. The conflict was resolved, and anxiety cleared.

Psychotherapy

Mohan knew about the odor coming out of his body. He didn't know the connection between the bad odor and masturbation. He was of the opinion that masturbation was wrong and it had spoiled his body. All these were in conscious mind. The connection between them (masturbation with semen discharge) was suppressed and was in the unconscious mind.

In psychotherapy he learnt that his feeling of body odor was his own feeling and nobody else felt it. He had to be educated as to the normal sexual instincts. This cleared his ignorance. This led to the further breakthrough in therapy. He believed those sexual acts had spoiled his body. When once he learnt that those acts were normal and do not cause any damage, he was relieved. He understood that his body was not damaged by his acts and hence no body odor was emanating from it. The ignorance was responsible for Mohan's problem and it was alleviated in psychotherapy. Mohan's problem is called neurosis. This is a very common problem in psychiatric practice.

Grief Reaction

A person called me over the phone and asked me for an emergency appointment. I asked him to come to my clinic. Two men came along with a girl. The girl looked dull. Her head was covered with a thick cloth. She had a blanket wrapped on her body. She was shivering. She was clenching her teeth. It appears she was suffering from fever. She was accompanied by her father and an uncle. Her father introduced her to me as Rajini of 11 years. I was a little concerned whether she was brought to me by mistake looking at the way she was wrapped with sheets. Her father reported she had been to many doctors and they had told she had no physical illness and advised a psychiatric consultation. I went through the treatment file and there was no indication of any physical illness. She had no relief from their treatment. Out of frustration she had alternative modes of treatment. Pilgrimages and worships didn't help. Her father was so much disturbed that he looked like a patient himself. He reported crying when alone and all of them were not even eating properly.

Rajini had abdominal pain, joints pain, back pain and headache. It was gradually increasing, and it was difficult for her father to see her agony. She would shiver as if she had fever. There was no relief from it with warm blanket. When she had abdominal pain she would fold her legs over her chest and squeezed her hands. Sometimes she had vomiting. Unable to bear the pain she had to toss in strange ways in bed. These attacks (it was their word) came in 8 to 10 attacks in a day. When she had joint pains, she was not able to move her limbs. She had generalized body weakness. When she had headache, she was holding her head tight and at times she had mildly banged her head to the wall. Her father was losing hopes and thought she would die. After all he was her father and his love for her made him not to lose his determination to get her cured.

I tried to find out if Rajini had disturbing incidents that could be responsible for her problems. Her mother suffered from some illness for four months and died about 2.5 months ago. Unable to withstand her mother's suffering from illness, the family felt it was better if her mother died. Rajini cried a lot after her death and was alright later. Approximately 15 days later Rajini's problems began. There were no other disturbing incidences. My examination of her didn't reveal any physical problem.

Rajini said she was disturbed about her mother's death, but gradually got over it. I asked her to remove the sheets covered on her head and body. Her father expressed her fever might increase. When she had no fever how it could increase. I explained to her shivering was not due to fever and it was because of anxiety. I said her problem was psychological and not to treat her as if she had a fever. I prescribed her antidepressant and antianxiety medicines. I asked her to come back after a week for psychotherapy sessions.

Rajini was brought back to me very next day. Her father said her trouble had increased and she was wrapped with blanket again. He said that everybody in the family was crying thinking something had happened to Rajini. I had to reassure her father that Rajini did not have any serious illnesses and not to worry so much. I convinced him with a great difficulty. I had given very small doses of medicines. I increased the medicines and sent her home with an advice for next therapy session after three days.

She was a little better after three days, but it was not to any significant extent. Her father was worried she was not alright even with 4 days treatment. Psychological problems are always slow to respond for the treatment. Her father got doubts whether her problem was psychological at all. He was of the opinion her problem was that of nerves. He asked me if she needed to consult a neurologist. I said that I was confident she did not need any neurological consultation.

Her father took her to a neurologist and learnt Rajini did not have any neurological problem. He apologized to me for taking her there against my opinion. I told him it was good and now he would not have any further doubts. A patient should be ready for the treatment and then only we can produce good results. Here her father's confidence was important because Rajini was a minor and entirely dependent on him. By the end of 4th session, they were ready for the treatment without any reservation. I sent her father out and spoke to Rajini alone. She denied of any worries at home or school. She denied about being upset very much about mother's death. I asked her how things were at home. Rajini became angry and began cursing most of the family. Her grandmother scolded her if she came late for the food. Her aunt (father's younger brother's wife who was in their joint family) was not so much loving to her as towards her own children. Her elder sisters scolded her for her stubbornness. She had no complaints on her father. She said he loved her, but he was out of the house most of the day (He had a business). She kept scolding all others in the family for about 15 minutes.

In the next session Rajini brought up a very interesting point. Sometimes she had noticed that her pains occurred after she was scolded. She revealed once again her problems with family members. She was a stubborn girl. If anybody scolded, she would refuse to eat and would shout. According to her father all loved Rajini. He could not understand Rajini's reaction towards others in the family. I learnt this was not Rajini's behavior earlier. One day her grandmother was serving food. The portion served was more than what Rajini wanted. Rajini became very angry. Her grandmother told her she could eat however much she could eat and to leave the rest. Rajini did not cool down. She refused to eat and walked away. Rajini said if her mother was there, she would have sat next to her and cajoled her to eat.

Another time her elder sister forgot to comb Rajini's hairs as the sister was getting late for the college. Rajini ranted and raved. In fact Rajini loved that sister. Rajini felt bad for her reaction. She cried and said " I don't know why I am doing like this. It is happening after the death of my mother." She said none of them matched her mother in caring. She cried again. She was studying in a convent school and was speaking well in English. Sometimes she said "sorry doctor I will not cry any more" I told her there was nothing wrong in crying and it was a normal feeling. The emotions should be expressed and not to be bottled up. The family members pointed towards her sister and would tell her to be like her sister and not to cry. If she cried in front of her father he would also start crying and she could not bear to see that. She tried to refrain from crying in front of her father for this reason. Sometimes after everybody slept, she would cry a lot in bed. I encouraged her not to suppress her crying. She began crying without control. When she became comfortable, she said if something was not alright with her the mother would sleep next to her. Food, clothes and all of her necessities were well taken care by her mother. The family members looked after her well, but it did not match her mother's care. How can anyone fill the void of her mother?

I asked her father to come inside and told him to let her cry. He said if she cried he could not control himself from crying. He did not want to make Rajini feel that he had lost his confidence. What is wrong in both crying together? If father cries, does it mean he is weak? Parents are also human beings. They have same feelings as others. There is nothing wrong in crying in front of the children, but they should not lose their confidence in life.

I was surprised to look at Rajini in the next session. She was nicely groomed and had worn nice clothes. Ins,tead of grumpy face there

Grief Reaction

was a smile. She reported her pains had reduced considerably. The whole session was spent on her description of how well her mother was taking care of her. In between she was crying, but the intensity of her crying had come down. Her attacks of pain had come down from 8 to 3 times per day. Before the attacks lasted for about 30 minutes and it reduced to about 10 minutes. Rajini accepted she was more upset about her mother's death than she realized. She accepted that when she was upset she was taking it out on others.

She had not accepted her mother's death fully. She was looking for others to fill that void. How can anyone fill the place of mother? Some fathers say, "I raised her without her mother and I am father and mother to her". He might have done some duties of her mother, but can anyone fulfill a mother's void.? People express like that, but no one can completely fill the void of another person. When a person is angry, he shouts. When Rajini shouted, others in the family shouted back at her. It was not possible for a younger person like Rajini to win against elders. The sick person demands extra attention and care. This seeking attention from the illness is called as secondary gain. Why her problem had decreased but had not gone fully?

Rajini's problem was not cured, even though she was aware of the reason, because sometimes the body gets adapted to it and it responds automatically in the same way as before. It is called as Pavlov's conditioning. The best example for this is jet lag that we experience when we go to another country like America. We experience sleep for a few days on arriving there in the day time (ours is night time here) rather than night time. Our body will have conditioned to our time and it needs a few days to adjust to their day and night. This some people call it as the function of body clock. In nervous system there is reticular activating system, which is responsible for this. Rajini's body had been conditioned to one behavior and pains. I had to decondition her with sedac (sedating current) treatment. It is not shock treatment. The patient is asked to think of the problem and a mild current is given to the head's temple regions. It causes an unpleasant feeling. The patient will associate this unpleasant feeling with his problem, and it makes the problem undesirable. Human being functions on pain pleasure principle. He avoids pain and seeks pleasure. In Rajini the unpleasant sensation from sedac treatment was stronger than her pains. This made her dislike the body pain and to come out of her problems. Rajini became alright. She began going to school. She had missed her school for quite some time. Despite missing school for many days, she passed in the examination. Her father came to inform me that Rajini had passed in the examination and had tears in his eyes, of course this time it was tears of happiness.

Her illness is called as grief reaction. It happens when a person experiences a very big loss like loss of a loved one, loss of a job, etc. usually it lasts from 4 to 6 weeks. It can last for six months also. It took longer because Rajini was young and anybody needs a mother at that age badly. Rajini could not express well because all were busy and nobody to listen to her. The internalized and unexpressed emotions took a toll on her. Rajini was treated with psychotherapy and deconditioning therapy.

Psychodynamics

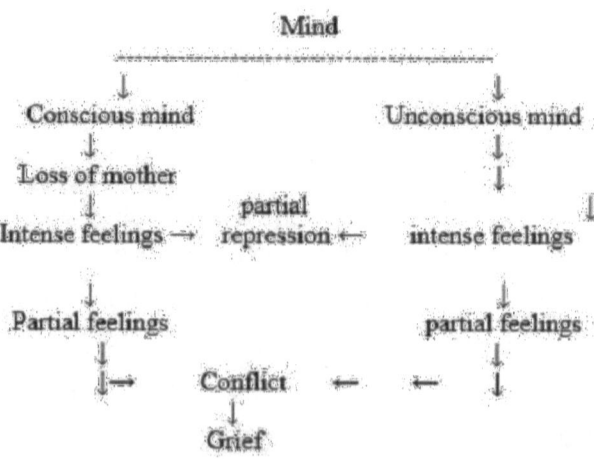

Rajini was depressed and upset about her mother's death a lot more than she realized. Her Ego repressed the feelings as there was no other possibility under the circumstances. She harbored the feelings of loss of her mother partially in both conscious and conscious minds. This resulted in conflict. She couldn't accept the loss completely. Her unconscious mind was trying to get the same affection from others as that from her mother. As it didn't work, it resulted in illness. The unconscious mind tried to get the same care through illness, and she was not getting it. She wouldn't reconcile. (secondary gain). This continuous conflict resulted in grief.

Psychotherapy

In psychotherapy she was made aware of her illness was not physical and it was psychological. She was informed that mind had different divisions conscious and unconscious parts. Her feeling of not getting the same affection as her mother from others was brought to her attention. This was because she was not reconciled to her mother's death. This was quite understandable as she was still at an age of needing mother intensely. She was taking it out of her feeling of loss of mother on others unintentionally. Being aware of these feelings her two parts of the mind stopped functioning oppositely. It resulted in psychological harmony and relief from her grief.

Gambling

Ramesh, a 35 years old man had headache, chest pain, limbs ache and general tiredness. He had poor sleep. He had taken treatment from his family doctor and had taken medications properly. His family doctor had told him that he had no physical illness and had given him some tonics for strength. His x ray, blood checkup, urine and stool examination reports were quite normal. Visiting temples and worships didn't give any relief. He had incurred quite a lot of expenditure for all the above reasons.

Ramesh was a successful steel vessels businessman in his town. Only his cousins were rivals in the town for this business. How can a person of this nature have any problem? He looked sad and anxious. He expressed that something was going on in the body and was worried something might happen to him. He was worried as to who would care for his family if something happened to him. He was afraid of even small aches. When he had chest pain he was afraid that he might die of heart attack. If he had headache, he thought that he might be having brain tumor. When he had weakness, he was afraid that he might get paralysis. If he had giddiness he was worried it might be high blood pressure. When his doctor declared that he had no physical problem, he would be alright for a while and would get some or the other physical symptom very soon.

He had a big file of all treatments and placed it before me. It was such a big file and I had to spend some time to view it. All tests and reports were normal. My examination also didn't reveal any physical illness. He was sad, otherwise looked alright. He denied of having any worries. I prescribed him an antidepressant and asked him to return for further treatment after a week.

He couldn't even wait for one week and came to see me in four days. He said that he didn't get any relief from the medication. I explained to him that antidepressants usually required 3 to 4 weeks to act. He was worried if something happened to him in the meanwhile who would care for his wife and children. All tests and consultations revealed that he had no physical problems and I questioned him where the question of danger to his life was. He agreed but expected that my medicines would give him immediate relief. He even doubted that I might have missed the diagnosis. He also thought that to appease him I might be telling that he had no physical problem. I had to assure him that I was not telling him just to satisfy him. I had to make him aware that his illness was there for three months and how it could be cured in 4 days.

Ramesh told me that he was suffering from this problem for two years and not for three months as reported earlier. He didn't reveal it as the family might get worried. I asked him to tell me all the worries that he had. He got puzzled. He had a firm belief that his problem was physical and I was asking him about his worries. He said that I had no idea about his problem and what his problem had to do with the worries. I had to explain the relationship between the mind and body and how worries can influence the body. A lot of physical symptoms have a root cause in mind.

In the 4th visit the discussion continued. Ramesh was stuck to his opinion that his problem was physical. He rejected again that worries could cause physical symptoms. He accused all doctors including me for not able to diagnose his problem. His accusation went on for about 15 minutes. I heard him without saying anything. At the end he asked me for my opinion. I told him that I was very aware of his problem, but he was not ready to accept that worries could cause physical symptom. I assured him that I was confident about my opinion. He expressed that somehow, he was beginning to have confidence in me. This indicated that he had partially agreed with what I had told. A psychiatrist has to look at each and every response in order to understand the patient and his problem. He accused me and other doctors for not diagnosing his problem. He would have not come for further appointments, if he really felt we were not in the right track. Why he didn't do this? This indicated that partially he had agreed with what I said and had confidence in me as well as other doctors. Then the question was why he was accusing me and other doctors? This was because he could not accept that it was psychological. We can sense the two parts of his mind here. Accepting the truth is always difficult. His forceful voice was in fact evidence for it rather than a rejection.

Ramesh came from an affluent family. He had a lot of ambitions in his life. All those ambitions were lost and he was even shy of facing his relatives. He was earning well in his business. He could save a lot of money after spending well for usual expenses. He went to a horse race two times. He was lucky and won well. As he earned easy money he was drawn into it. He made it a habit. When he won in the race he would add some more money into it and bet high again in order to make more money. This went on for two years and it had increased in one year. He lost track of how much was invested and how much was lost. When he realized he had lost all of his savings.

He didn't reveal to anyone about his involvement in horse race and losses. His wife and parents had immense confidence in him. His race habit continued. Often he closed his shop and went for horse racing. This kept increasing. When he closed his shop for the race, he lied to the family that he was going to the bigger town for health checkup. In the beginning the family didn't even doubt him. The truth had to come out sooner or later. The family came to know about his race habit. The business had also come down because of frequent closures of the shop. The parents advised him to stop from going to races. Somehow or the other secretly he would go to the races. He had to close the shop because of it was in losses. A highly profitable business was under loss and had to be closed. He was ashamed to go out as he had lost his reputation. He sold his house and moved to another town and rented a house. He lost further the money he had from selling his house also in races.

In the next visit I asked him why he shouldn't stop races and start a business in the new town. He said that his cousins had advanced very well in the same business and there was no way he could catch up with them. He and his cousins were rivals in business all along. These cousins always had a better business than him and were more rich also. He was jealous of them and wanted to overtake them in business. He couldn't overtake them. He thought of making quick money in racing and thus could overtake them. Ramesh didn't give up races involvement. He wanted to make a lot of money in race again. He strongly believed that he would be able to make big money in it.

Everybody has to live his own life. One should not be jealous and try to make life a competition. There was no way to make easy money. One can come up only by hard work. One should live according to their own possible means. All these had an impact on Ramesh and he promised that he will stop going to races. He wanted to start the same business in the new place.

Ramesh came for the next visit on the following week. I was taken aback about what he said. He was left with 50,000.00 Rupees. He wanted to put all that money into races and try for his luck for the last time. One can imagine the gravity of the bad effect of gambling. I asked him if he lost all that money again and became broke what he would do? He told me that I had a pessimistic attitude. I told him that he should be realistic and think what he would do if he lost all the money. As per his own experience he had lost a whole lot of money and had won only a little. I told him he should believe in his business acumen rather than races. I even told him not to gamble in races. Of course, I could not stop him, I could only suggest him. The decision was up to him. I made this clear to him.

I had no contact from him for one month. When he came he was more cheerful. He told me that he had stopped going to races. He had started a steel vessel business with the money he had. The business was picking up slowly. He stopped comparing himself with his cousins. He said that he had learnt a big lesson in his life and would continue in this path. He lost the desire to make quick money. He returned to see me after a year. He had brought a thank you card for me. He reported that he was involved in his business and it had improved more than he expected. He said that he would never venture into any gambling. His family was also happy.

Human being is basically greedy and wants to make quick money. This greed draws people to gambling. Generally, in gambling losses are more than the winnings. When they win some time, the people get drawn into it. It becomes a habit. We can say the above characteristics are that of a gambling personality. There are people going to races in a limited way and have not lost the property or the family. They use it as a hobby and not for making money. In other words, anything in a limited manner is not harmful.

Psychodynamics

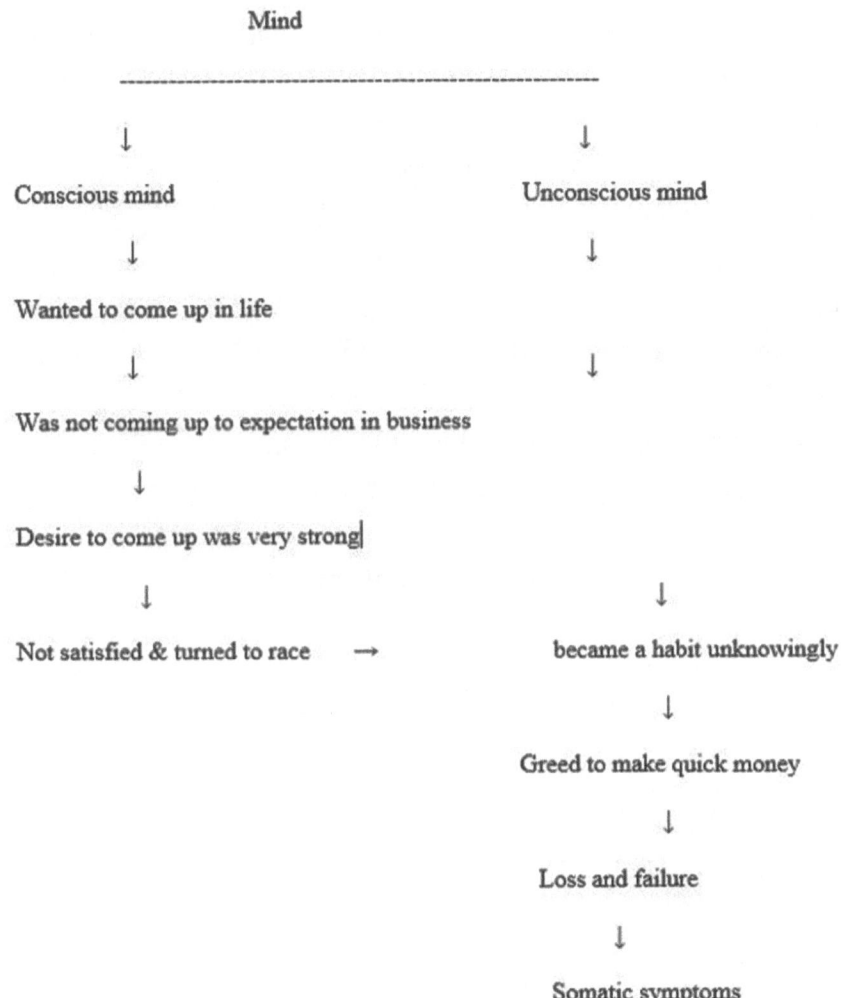

Ramesh's wanting to come up in life and dissatisfaction of his achievement turned life into a competition. His earnings in business was not enough to overtake his cousins. It turned unconsciously to horse racing habit to make quick money. His conscious mind was not approving this. The resulting conflict caused his problem.

Psychotherapy

Ramesh learnt in psychotherapy that he had no physical problem and his problem was psychological. It was brought to his awareness that there was no evidence for the presence of any physical illness. It was difficult to make him accept. He had made life a competition to overtake his cousins. When he could not achieve it in business, he turned to horse racing to make quick money. He lost the money and a good business. He realized horse racing had become a habit. He realized that he couldn't make quick money in racing and yet wouldn't leave it, because it had become a habit. He was not satisfied with what he was, because of his expectation to overtake his cousins. He understood being satisfied with what he was important for a happy life. He reconciled not to make life a competition. He concluded that he had to learn to enjoy life within his means. He learnt to be happy and satisfied.

Selfishness

Reshma, aged 34 years came to me saying that she was overwhelmed with some problems. She was physically alright. She had severe headache for some time. She said that she had become a nervous wreck. She had poor sleep. She would become restless often. Her husband recently had moved to USA. She had stayed here along with her two daughters because of they were in the middle of school year. After their examinations all of them were to join her husband in USA. To wind up everything here and to go to USA she had a lot of things to be taken care of. This she felt it was very draining and overwhelming.

She had inherited a land and was able to sell for a huge amount. She wanted to avoid paying taxes on the income from selling the property by investing in another property (as per the legal provision). She had to consult a lawyer for this. Her husband had a flat, which had to be renovated for giving it for rent. She had to find a reliable tenant. She had to make arrangement for collection of rents. If a tenant leaves she had to make arrangement for renovation and find a new tenant. There was no body to look after these things after she moved to USA. Her only brother refused to take care of all these things. She had to take care of all the above before going to USA.

She thought of finding a property management company to take care of all these things. They were demanding a huge price, which she was not ready to pay. She talked to her husband over the phone and he suggested her to do whatever she thought was best. She had to take care of the children and their studies amidst these. Her husband couldn't come here to take care of all these things, because it was a new job and would not get any permission. She felt that she was going "nuts" (her own description). She was a homemaker and never took care of such things. Her husband was taking care of all such things. She was unable to decide one way or the other. My psychiatric evaluation revealed anxiety, otherwise alright. I sent her with a recommendation that she might need a couple of psychotherapy sessions. She was given a small dose of antianxiety agent, which she refused to take.

She promptly came for the next two psychotherapy sessions. Again, a run over of all of her problems took place. I asked her what the problem was as she could figure out. She said that she was not able to decide and sometimes her mind would go blank. She had to take care of all these things in about 20 days and she had already booked tickets to USA. The mind was going blank added to the problem and the time available was short. I agreed with her that she had so many things to take care of in a short time. Property matters are time consuming and she was expecting too much in a short time. She didn't want to sell the flat because of taxes involved. Giving the property for rent also involved a lot of problems. She wanted to keep the house property and had to invest the money that she got from inheritance without paying taxes and didn't want headaches of renting out the flat. I pointed out this to her that she wanted to get all the things done without losing any money. She agreed.

Her contention was why she should pay taxes. I asked her if there was a way that she can attain all these things as she wanted in a limited period. She admitted that she had shouldered a big responsibility didn't think of any way. The principle of life is if you want something you have to give up something. Human being is very selfish and wants to get the best of all without giving up anything. Here she had to decide either to sell, pay taxes and be happy without the headaches of managing it or to keep all of them and take troubles associated with it. This was the conflict. She was undecided about it. She should think pros and cons of both and come to a decision. Ultimately it boiled down to deciding. Inability to decide is known as aboulomania.

The question arose in my mind why she was so rigid and hard on herself. Our personal character formation begins with parents. Our first woman in life is mother and first man in life is father. Their relationship to the baby pretty much determines the way we are going to react with future men and women in life. The extended family members, teachers, etc also will influence further our personality character. As a result of all we develop unique personality nature. If we know a person very well we can almost predict how he is going to react in a given situation. We tend to react in our own unique way on any task. That is exactly the reason we seek somebody else's opinion on an important task. Being a different person with different nature he may suggest something, which we could not think because of our unique personality nature.

My further exploration revealed that Reshma's parents were self-made, hardworking, disciplined, time bound and with no procrastination in their tasks. It had an impact on her. I asked her whether there was any other possible solution to this problem. She didn't think of any other possibility to it. I asked her did she have to take care of all these tasks in such a short time and in such matters of extreme urgency might be bad. I told her that peace of mind is very important in whatever decision she took. One may have to forego something for the sake of one's mental peace. I also brought to her notice that normal selfishness was alright, but what was the use of it, if it disturbed her peace of mind. There was no other way but to make a hard decision. Not deciding could cause even more disturbance of mind.

I told her again to peacefully think of any other possibility and not to close the option by saying that there was no option. She was brought up by parents with strict values as stated above. She had inculcated them. I raised a point whether it was necessary for her to finish all these in 20 days? After I raised this matter she said that she could keep status quo on all these matters and go to USA. After settling there for a couple of months she could come back and take care of all the matters, meanwhile she could seek the opinion of her husband also while in USA. She decided that was her final decision. After she decided she was relieved and got good sleep also.

Psychodynamics

Patients have high expectation on psychiatrists. They think that he is next to god and has easy solution for everything. There are realistic problems for which there are only realistic solutions. A psychiatrist will never give any solution to the problem. He will only help the patient to arrive at a solution. Reshma was in a situation never like this before. She was a housewife. Earlier her parents and later her husband would take care of everything in the family. Suddenly she was faced with a situation of investing her inherited money from property, renting out their flat with all renovations, finding a new tenant and care for all the things like children's examination and to run the family. She was brought up in a much-disciplined family and to take care of everything without procrastinating. She was also selfish and didn't want to lose any money for taxes and not to spend much for renovation. The time that she had was short. She knew consciously the conflicts involved. She was bent upon finishing all these things before going to USA. Unconsciously she knew it was impossible. She didn't admit it because of her strong superego, which refused procrastination. This resulted in conflict leading to all the symptoms as above.

Psychotherapy

She was made aware that she was overwhelmed with problems. She was a house- wife suddenly in a situation to handle several things in a short time. She had a strong superego and hated any procrastination. Her aim to take care of all the matters in 20 days was too much for anybody. Because she was bent upon taking care of all of them in a short time her mind could not think of another alternative. She learnt that she could postpone some decisions for a couple of months, and it gave relief to her. When once she made the decision to postpone the decision, her stress was less. Her decision to postpone the decision gave her an opportunity to discuss with her husband. It gave some mental strength (anybody prefers a second opinion from a close person on very difficult problems). In this decision she got more time to take care of things after settling in USA. After this I had no contact with her. I do not know whether she came back and took care of all tasks. I hope that she is alright.

Cramps

There is a lot of ignorance and stigma about mental disorder or illness. The opinion amongst people is that any physical symptom felt in the body ought to be physical. Psychological means it is either a lie or it is imaginary is the concept prevailing amongst public. More than 50% of all real physical symptoms are deep rooted in mind. Our conscious and unconscious minds can command through the brain to cause real physical symptoms like cramps, pain, etc in any part of the body. As described in other chapters whenever there is a conflict between the different parts of the mind there is generation of anxiety. Our three parts of the mind can be compared to a court. In a court there is a complainant, a defendant and a judge. The judge gives a judgment. If the judge is weak what a chaos it causes in court. If our ego is weak, it is like a weak judge in the court and it causes chaos in mind. The chaos causes mental turmoil and leads to all types of psychological problems. Usually an individual with well-developed ego resolves his conflicts within a reasonable time. Sometimes the conflicts are so strong, and ego is not strong enough, it may result in a chaotic situation and make him indecisive. Prolonged conflict with indecisiveness can lead to psychological problems. Our brain doesn't decide anything, it is our mind which decides and commands for action through the brain. Brain is actually like a faithful servant of our mind. If the conflict between conscious and unconscious minds is not resolved, a confused mind sends confused messages to brain and it results in a confused action in the body.

When I was with a group of friends there was a casual discussion on cramps of the body. The opinion of all of them was that it was a physical problem and not even one mentioned it could be psychological also. I opened the Pandora by saying cramps can be psychological also. It raised some commotion. Some friends agreed and most of them disagreed. Our meeting ended that way. One friend called me the next day and asked if I could help someone that he knew. He told me that they were desperate.

He sent the patient to my clinic. Rama, a 14 yrs. old girl was accompanied by her mother. Rama had attacks of cramps with pain in her waist. Several doctors said she was physically alright, but her agony continued. She was taken to all types of specialist doctors and even alternative medical specialists like ayurvedic homeopathic, etc. She was taken to even black magic specialists and curse removers, etc. This kind of approach is not unusual in our society. Almost all of our patients will have undergone all types of treatments before coming to a psychiatrist. Her family was fed up of Rama's problem. It had a large financial drain on the family. Her father was a schoolteacher with a limited income. The parents had lost hope. At this stage my friend suggested my name. It came as a silver lining in a dark cloud. She was not taken to any psychiatrist, because it never occurred to them and nobody had suggested also.

Rama came with clean clothes. She had vermillion (red dot on the forehead worn usually by Hindus) on her forehead. She was well groomed. Her actions revealed that she was a very active girl. The attacks of cramps with pain began on the waist while taking bath 2 years ago and worsened in the last 3 months. It was not continuous but came in attacks. Lately she was getting attacks about 20 times a week. It was intense pain with cramps. She kept describing them as attacks. During the attacks sometimes she just stared blindly for a few seconds. Some other times she would spit saliva on her hand and smeared on her face. After the attack she went to sleep for about 10 minutes. When she had attacks, she was observed to be in a kind of fear. She had records of various doctors ruling out of any physical illness. These types of attacks can be due to a kind of neurological seizures (epilepsy) also. A mere physical examination doesn't reveal any defect in real epilepsy cases. Hyperventilation induces seizure in real epilepsy. I subjected her to this test. I asked her to continue taking deep breaths for 6 minutes. It didn't induce any attacks. If it is seizures of central nervous system problem, hyperventilation for even 2 to 3 minutes will induce an attack. The thematic apperception test revealed that she was a very angry person and she wanted to be number one in everything. She was advised to see me for psychotherapy sessions.

One week later her mother brought her and said that her illness had worsened and cried. I had to comfort her by saying Rama's problem of 2 years could not be solved in one or two weeks and she had to be treated for a longer time. Besides this ups and downs is natures making and illnesses also go through ups and downs. Her mother seemed to understand this and I sent her out and talked to Rama. I tried to find out from Rama if she was upset on anything and what circumstances had led to this. She denied any upsetting incidents. I delved into what all she did in that week. I learnt that one day she wanted to go to a party with her friends and mother refused permission because of the fear that Rama might get an attack and her illness might become public. This may cause difficulty in her marriage chances in future (In many societies an unmarried girl with illness has to face rejection by the prospective bridegrooms). Following mother's denying the permission she had 3 attacks. At that time her mother even felt guilty that she didn't allow her to go and even thought attacks might have not happened if she had permitted her to go.

Treatment continued with weekly therapy sessions. Another time Rama asked her father for money to buy something. Her father refused to give money saying it was not necessary. Following this she had an attack. At this stage I had to reassure her mother that her illness was not serious one and not to be afraid so much. I also suggested her to downplay the reactions whenever Rama had attacks. A psychiatrist must deal with others concerned also, whenever necessary. Rama's frustration and dejection continued. She asked me to give her something to die. She said she was not needed by anybody. Her parents were so much loving and asked her why she felt like not being needed. She admitted that they loved her. She said that her parents were more worried about her problem becoming known to others. For my question of whether it was wrong on the part of her parents to feel that way, she had no response. I asked her whether it was alright for her, if it became public. She also said that she didn't want it to be public. At this stage she felt unhappy for being angry on her parents for this reason. In one week, she had 20 attacks and out of them we had a definite indication in 5 attacks to feel the attacks occurred whenever she was upset. I have not described all the circumstances in which attacks happened. All of them had occurred in similar circumstances. I pointed out to Rama in details how her attacks were related to getting upset about something or other.

Her father's financial position was not very good as mentioned earlier. She was to see me for a session one day and she asked her father for money. Her father refused to give her money without even finding out what for she wanted. She gathered all small changes she had with her and she came. I was very happy about it as it showed her strong motivation to get better. She didn't have an attack also, which was a very positive development. I told her that she should not get upset whenever she was denied of something. She should try to see if she could achieve it in some other way like this time, if it was so important and reasonable. I even appreciated her for her very mature and appropriate behavior at that stage. She expressed that her parents were upset about her illness and she felt bad for making her parents unhappy.

In the following sessions many things became apparent. Rama hated to hear "no" from anyone and for anything. When denied something she would get extremely upset. In the last 5 attacks (only circumstances of 2 attacks have been described) she had been related to denial of something. She reluctantly agreed. As stated above she wanted to be first always. She should be first for her parents love also. I raised the issue if parents loved her siblings did it mean that parents didn't love her? Human being can love many people at the same time, where is the question of more or less? Rama loved both of her parents and she couldn't even say whom she loved more. She agreed and even felt bad for her silly behavior (she described it like this). I consoled her by saying that she was young and there was a lot to learn in life yet. Her reaction was not uncommon at all. At this stage she recalled that she had some attacks whenever she felt parents expressed love towards her siblings.

She was very angry natured and was very angry when her parents were unable to satisfy her material needs. Her father was a middle-class person and financially limited. He had to manage the family within his means. I asked Rama if she knew anyone who got all he wanted. This is life. All of us get only some things and not all. This is the truth of life. We should learn to be happy for what we get and accept with bitterness what we don't get. She, in fact thanked me for opening her knowledge about life. She was also a part of the family and had to understand the difficulties of running the family. Her demands should be affordable for the family. She agreed. It was pointed out to her that she was unknowingly trying to get what she wanted through illness. It was also a fact that parents have to treat children differently for various reasons like age, circumstances, illness, etc, etc, eg: two years elder sister's needs may be different than that of an younger sister. It is not a discrimination, but the needs are different at different ages. If a sibling is not well he requires more care at that time. These are facts of life. She seemed to take all these things in good spirit. Rama's illness served the purpose of demanding more attention from parents.

At this stage I was quite well aware of Rama's illness. My treatment had a positive effect. Her attacks had reduced from 20 per week to about 5 per week, but had not stopped. In spite of so much therapy why her problem was not cured?. Here we have to understand that her body and mind were adapted to the illness. Our body and mind will get adapted to good or bad things unknowingly. This we call as conditioning. I decided to subject her to deconditioning therapy. I subjected her to SEDAC treatment. In this I asked Rama to remember her attacks and passed a small current to her temples through a treatment machine. This is not the same as Shock treatment (electro convulsive therapy). Sedac is given in a conscious state and anesthesia is not given. The current is just enough to make the patient feel unpleasant while thinking of attacks.. Gradually mind starts associating attacks with the unpleasant stimulus and makes it undesirable. This is called deconditioning therapy. This is based on Pavlov's conditioning theory.

Pavlov demonstrated like this. He proposed that a neutral stimulus can be made to be a positive stimulus. He demonstrated on a dog. He rang the bell and measured the stomach acidity in the dog, there was no increase in the stomach acidity. Next he rang the bell and gave food, there was increase in acidity. After repeatedly doing like he just rang the bell without giving food, still there was increase in acidity. The dog had associated bell with food. Here neutral stimulus became a positive stimulus. This he labeled it as conditioning response. In Sedac the same principle is used for deconditioning.

Pavlov's conditioning theory

He demonstrated on dog.

1. Rang the bell → no increase in acidity
2. Rang the bell + food → increase in acidity

    After a few times

3. Rang the bell without food → increase in acidity

A neutral stimulus (bell) had become a positive stimulus.

After a few Sedac treatments Rama was free of attacks. The question here is whether Rama was faking the problem? In fact her parents had raised this question to me. She was definitely not lying. A lying person will not have strain on his face. He will not bother about his illness and even doesn't participate in treatment properly. He will not do anything to deprive him of what he enjoys to do. His attacks happen in different circumstances at different times. Rama's cure was achieved in 8 psychodynamic psychotherapy sessions and 4 sedac treatments.

Psychodynamics

Her ID's (refer to mind mystery chapter) instinctual drive was narcistic (selfish and wanted more love from the parents). Her material needs were not met by parents for financial constraints. This remained in her unconscious mind. However, her parents were not happy about it. A child incorporates parental values (superego). The resulting conflict ID and superego was not resolved. It resulted in anxiety and in turn resulted in attacks. Her ego (partly not matured enough, in a 14 yrs old girl) was not able to solve. Being unaware of the conflict her ID mind wanted to fulfill her desires anyway. Her superego was unhappy with the ID's attitude.

Psychotherapy

In psychotherapy understanding of her ID's instinctual desires (narcissistic) and the conflict with her superego was brought to her awareness. The awareness of longing to be first and not understanding of the reality like her parent's financial position, etc also helped her. Unconsciously she was trying to satisfy her narcissistic needs by her behavior. Her superego hated her narrow and narcissistic behavior. This conflict was explored and it helped her to accept and then change her behavior. When ID (ID is mostly in unconscious mind) became conscious there was no conflict. Absence of conflict meant there was no anxiety. She became more peaceful in her mind. Psychodynamic psychotherapy was carried out to remove the root cause of the problem.

She was completely alright and had no attacks for one month. In the next 3 months I discontinued her medicines gradually. Believe it or not in our next meeting in the same group of friends my friend (who sent Rama) was the first to say physical symptoms can be a cause of deep rooted psychological problems. Here the question arises why her problem was not solved by just giving sedac treatment alone. Sedac treatment is a symptomatic treatment. If only sedac treatment was given her problem would have relapsed after some time, because the root cause of the problem was not treated.

Allergy

I had just returned from USA with an intention to serve my own country and people. I was apprehensive about my practice. It was prevailing in the society that there was no medicine and cure for mental illness. This was reflected in news, articles, sayings and movies. This was because of ignorance and stigma about mental illness. People were not consulting a psychiatrist, unless it was severe and unmanageable. For mild and moderate problems they were not seeking treatment. They were used to seek refuge in worships, charlatans (quacks), black magicians, spiritual healers, etc.

I was surprised when I received a call from a doctor requesting me to treat his patient. He was a very reputed family physician and Kiran was his patient. Kiran had allergy and was not responding to usual allergy treatment by allergists. When he suggested for consultation with me there was a big emotional outburst in Kiran's family. Some of his relatives were angry with him and suggested that Kiran should be taken to another doctor. Kiran' family had been to other doctors already and even allergists. They knew there was no point in getting another opinion. They decided to bring him to me. Kiran had allergy problem, which was not cured by any doctors. The doctor had read somewhere that allergy could be caused by psychological problems also and hence he referred him to me.

Kiran was 31 years old, mild mannered person talked with a smile in spite of his agony. It was obvious that he was putting on a smile with great difficulty. He was dejected about his allergy. It began about 2 years prior to consultation. He did not report any incident that could have triggered allergy. It began in the area of his wearing of spectacles. Gradually it had spread to the whole body. He would get allergy in attacks. First he would have itching and then eruption of rashes. After rashes subsided the skin became dark. This black color of skin would clear in a couple of hours. Sometimes he had intense itching, rashes and discoloration of the skin; it was painful for others to see him.

He had seen allergy and skin specialists with no avail. All types of tests were done. He was even given corticosteroids and allergy medicines. His allergy didn't respond at all. In the beginning corticosteroids helped him for a while but relapsed later. More and more corticosteroids had to be given to maintain the improvement. Corticosteroids should not be given like that. The doctor got frightened of his corticosteroids treatment. Kiran had stopped using soaps, terilene (a kind of synthetic) clothes and leather slippers as per the advice of the doctors. He was using soap nut powder for bath and wore cotton clothes as per the advice of the doctors. Nothing seemed to help. Sometimes he had noticed his allergy had increased when he was upset. At that stage I didn't have any clue to say there was a connection between allergy and psychological factors in Kiran. He denied of any worries. His appetite, sleep, etc were normal.

Kiran came from a poor family. Even the family had difficulty for adequate food. After he finished his studies he had difficulty in getting a job. He had thought of suicide, being frustrated about unemployment. Finally he got a job in Bangalore and brought his parents and siblings to Bangalore. He helped his siblings for their education. He earned a good name as a worker in a factory. He was friendly to his colleagues. Someone suggested that his allergy would go if he got married. His parents arranged for his marriage. The allergy didn't disappear even after 10 months of marriage. He had stated that sometimes allergy increased when he was upset. Thematic

Apperception Test revealed that he had a lot of bottled up anger. A lot of people have this kind of nature and one cannot say that could be the reason for his allergy.

Being uncertain about the root cause of his problem, I subjected him for hypnosis. In olden days hypnosis was popular and in wide usage. The effect of hypnosis is short lived and because of this reason hypnosis was abandoned as treatment. Even now people carry out hypnosis in front of audience and it is a fascinating show to people. Even now hypnosis is carried on in short lived stresses, like war neurosis. Here I had used Hypnosis to find out the deep rooted problem of Kiran. About 50% of the people cannot be hypnotized even if they completely cooperate. Patient's cooperation is important here. He should have a good concentration for hypnosis. Kiran was a good candidate for hypnosis as he had good concentration and was fully cooperative. It was very successful.

In hypnosis I asked him to concentrate on one thing and follow my instructions properly. He was brought to semiconscious state. When he lost his control on conscious mind I began questioning him. About two years ago kiran's brother hit their younger sister for not bringing the clothes given for pressing(ironing). Kiran was very fond of this sister. Kiran became very angry with that brother. Without shouting or saying anything he just bottled up his anger. Allergy began for the first time. His parents always sided towards his younger brother in any disputes. They would blame Kiran rather than his younger brother. He admitted that whenever he became very angry and couldn't express he would get allergy. I learnt quite a lot in hypnosis about his problem. He was still under hypnosis and I suggested him that he will not have allergy for any reason. I also instructed him to drink water and should wash his face with soap after he came out of hypnosis. Then I brought him out of hypnosis. He slowly opened his eyes and drank water and washed his face with soap and he didn't have allergy. I sent him home with instructions to use all the things as before the start of allergy.

A few days later kiran had allergy again. I had to treat him with hypnosis again. Hypnosis effect doesn't last long. Because of this reason hypnotic treatment was abandoned. The hypnosis is carried out in unconscious state. Psychotherapy is carried out in conscious state and it is lasting. I hypnotized him again to give him immediate relief. After this I asked him to come for psychotherapy sessions. The weekly sessions continued for 11 weeks. In those 11 weeks Kiran had allergy attacks four times and out of these two were somewhat severe attacks. I tried to ascertain the circumstances of his attacks. Kiran was not aware of them consciously. The mind tries to block it from coming to the conscious level. This is called as repression. Because of this if we ask the patient about the reason, he would not know the reason consciously. Some times our attempt to explore will not give any results. We should put together all the pieces of information like that in a puzzle in order to get the answer.

I told Kiran nothing happened without any reason. There must be very strong hidden reason behind this allergy. I asked him to think of everything that might upset him before the attack of allergy. At that time he said that he had a letter from his wife, who was in her parent's place. He said there was nothing unusual in it. He also said that because I told him to think of the circumstances, he just told me. He told me if he didn't say anything I might feel bad and hence he said it. A psychiatrist should be very vigilant and patient. The thought in my mind was did he really say it to please me? or was he dragging me unconsciously to something? Sometimes we consider such incidences as usual and leave it. Somehow I felt that he was trying unconsciously to communicate something to me. I asked him casually how his wife was. She had written a letter asking him to take her back into his house. I told him jovially that probably she missed him. He also missed her. She was 6 months pregnant. He said his wife and his parents didn't get along well. His parents had told him clearly not to bring her back or else to move out of the house. He was torn between the two as to what to do. He believed moving to a new house when the woman was pregnant was a bad omen. His wife was repeatedly writing letters for the same. Even if he moved to a new house she had to go back to her parents for the delivery. She would be in the new house for just 2 months. He was angry on his wife that she wanted him to spend so much money for the sake of 2 months and could not wait for 2 months. He was angry on his parents because they had told him clearly not to bring back her into their house. He was bearing the expenditure of the family and even then the parents were asking him to move to a different house. He begged his parents to tolerate his wife just for 2 months till the delivery and then he would move to a new house, for which parents refused. He was angry and frustrated about the impossible situation he was in. Then only itching and rashes began this time. He decided to ask an uncle of his wife to advise her to stay with her parents till the delivery. I raised a point that whether his bottled up anger could be responsible for his allergy. He agreed for it. He felt bad that he was unable to solve the problem and depended upon his wife's uncle for solving the problem. I raised question as to what he would do if her uncle couldn't solve it. Kiran said that he would tell his wife to stay back with her parents till delivery and leave it like that. He acted accordingly and his allergy disappeared.

Another time he had an allergy attack. I had instructed him to keep track of circumstances leading to the attacks of allergy. His uncle's family took him away in the middle of the night to help them in solving a problem. His uncle got drunk and had a fight with some people. Kiran intervened and was taking his uncle to leave him to his house. On the way those people attacked Kiran and his uncle.

Kiran developed some bleeding injuries. He was able to get away from the attackers and went to police station to file a complaint against the attackers. The attackers had already filed a complaint against him and Kiran had to stay in jail. He was released the next day when the police came to know that Kiran was innocent. Kiran got immensely angry on his uncle for his drinking and getting him into this predicament. I could easily sense how angry he was while talking about it. After he expressed the anger his allergy subsided. I analyzed other situations of his allergic attacks. Myself and Kiran came to the conclusion that he had attacks of allergy whenever he had bottled up anger. Anger should not be bottled up, instead it should be expressed in a mature and socially acceptable way. Bottled up anger will always causes problem. Gradually with the adoption of expressing anger Kiran's allergy attacks came down and eventually he was free from it completely. He was able to use soaps, terilene clothes,etc as before.

The question may arise in the minds of readers whether all allergies are psychological. Some allergies are because of real physical problem. Then how to assess whether the allergy is physical or psychological? Indeed it is a very tough and challenging question even for a specialist. If allergy is physical it can be detected by various tests, which can identify the exact allergen (material responsible for allergy). The mind can be a culprit also. It has been proven in laboratories. In a famous experiment 8 people were taken by Ikemi and others for this purpose. These 8 people were allergic to a particular kind of leaves. They were not allergic to chestnut leaves. They blindfolded these 8 people and made them touch the allergenic leaves saying it was not chestnut leaves. They didn't get allergy attacks. Then they made them touch chestnut leaves saying they were allergenic leaves and they developed allergy. This demonstrated the role of mind in allergy.

In many people with allergy there is not a definite allergen responsible for allergy. In such cases there is a strong possibility of psychological factors being responsible. Witkower and engel studied 90 people with allergy and assessed their life circumstances and found out in 77 people some psychological incidence was responsible for allergy attacks. Mind is a wonder. The more we know about it the more we know about its influence on the body.

Psychodynamics

Kiran was a mild mannered person. He was not expressing anger and instead bottled up the anger. He had developed a typical personality nature. Any feelings when not expressed may cause problems. He suppressed his anger and it found expression unconThis resulted in conflict between the two parts of his mind. In conscious mind the anger was suppressed and in unconscious mind it had found expression in allergy.

Psychotherapy

Social stigma against mental illness had to be dealt with at first. Mental problem didn't mean madness was the first thing to be dealt with. Kiran had to be educated that mind was not one entity and it had different parts like conscious and unconscious minds. He was not used to express anger. The bottled up anger acted through unconscious mind resulting in psychological conflict. This conflict found expression in body i.e. skin. He had to be made aware of the relationship between the mind and body. He was made aware of his unconscious mind by revealing what was elicited under hypnosis. When the unconscious mind became conscious mind there was no longer any conflict. When there was no conflict there was no anxiety and thus his allergy also cleared. After learning this he began expressing anger in a more appropriate manner.

Fear of Devil

Suma was 24 years old college young lady. She was shy and sensitive from the beginning. She was not good in mingling with people. She had no friends. Books were her friends. She was labeled as book worm by her college mates. She was a first rank student every year. Because of her scholastic achievement she was a pet for the parents and teachers. Who doesn't like an obedient and well studying young lady? Parents thought that sometimes she should have been born as a boy, because she was excellent in studies. One night Suma shouted that someone was trying to kill her. Parents felt she was dull for about 15 days prior to this and opined that she was just tired. Parents assured her that no one could come inside and told her not to be afraid. She began saying it many times that her life was in danger and there was a big plot to kill her. She was not allowing anybody to come nearer her except parents and siblings. If anyone came home and went near her she would start scolding them saying they were trying to kill her. Parents were concerned but they thought she would be alright after a while. They didn't want to talk to anybody for the fear of being labeled as mad.

One month elapsed. Suma began laughing and talking inappropriately. She quit eating claiming the food was poisoned. She was not sleeping enough for the fear of someone coming to kill her. She began claiming that she heard some voices. Sometimes she would hear voices of deceased people also. She claimed the voice was her deceased uncle's voice. She feared that devils were trying to kill her. One day a postman came to deliver a mail and she chased him away saying he had come to kill her. The neighbors came out for her shouting. They began saying that she was possessed by a devil. On that day parents decided to do something and not to leave it anymore.

Some well- intentioned relative suggested a spiritual healer saying she was possessed by devil. The healer chanted some mantras and repeatedly sprinkled water on her face saying " Mohini go away". He branded her with hot iron. He hit her with a broom. He said that he would burn the devil in fire. He collected his hefty fees, but Suma remained the same. Someone suggested her stars were not alright and made parents perform some worships and made them give charity. They went on pilgrimage and made offerings to god as per the suggestions of some more. They took her to a spiritual guru (monk). None of them helped. After all known possibilities were over they were lost and someone suggested them to take her to a psychiatrist.

At first only father came to see me. He explained all the problems. He said that Suma refused to come to me. He asked me what he could do ? Suma was close to her maternal uncle and I suggested him to get that uncle to advise her to see me. It worked and the father brought her to me. Suma refused to see me alone. She didn't let me close the door and shouted "don't close the door. You are trying to kill me". She shouted like this for about 5 minutes. Father felt ashamed of her behavior towards me. He thought that she was disrespecting me. He tried to stop her and advised her to behave properly. I advised her father not to intervene and let everything to me. Suma continued to shout. Only in a very mild manner I told her that I was not going to kill her. I wanted to help her as a doctor. Suma said that everyone ran away from her and why I was not scared?. I told her that both of us needn't be scared of each other. At that point I introduced myself as Dr. Druva Kumar and was trying to help her as a psychiatrist.

I even told her that she was scolding me with a fear that I would kill her. I told her that I was there to help her. Suma laughed and said" I am not mad and you are mad". I told her that I had never said that she was mad. I told her that I didn't know her problem and I was just trying to figure it out. I told her my evaluation was not even complete and how could I label her as mad? This had some effect on her. She began crying profusely. She told me not to come nearer her and she wanted to talk to me from a distance. I agreed for that. For the first time she began talking to me with respect. I tried to elicit what bothered her and was not successful in my effort. She was still looking at me with suspicion. At such times we have to make the patient comfortable. I tried to find out her interests and came to know that she was a stamp collector. I asked her about her latest collection. She went on describing for about half an hour. The session ended that way. I told her that I would like to see her again and gave her an appointment myself, instead of sending her to my receptionist. She liked my personal interest.

Suma was more comfortable and she agreed to talk to me alone, but asked me to keep the door open in the next visit. She expressed that she heard three voices talking between themselves telling "she should be killed". She also heard voices of her deceased uncle and grandmother telling her "come to us". She arrived at the conclusion that it must be their devils (There is a feeling in the society a deceased person may become a devil) voice. During the nights if there were any sounds, she would think they were devil's voices. She believed that food was poisoned and hence she quit eating. If anyone passed in front of their house she felt they were going to kill her. If she found two people talking she thought they were trying to hatch a plot to eliminate her. Instead of suffering so much, often she thought of hanging herself and die. I ascertained that she didn't have any physical problems and suggested her to be admitted to our hospital. Suma refused to be admitted saying she had no illness. Her contention was that she was targeted by devils and why she should be admitted, at least I was able to convince her to take medicines. I prescribed her some antipsychotic medicines and sent her home. She agreed to take medicines. In a hospital we can give treatment more aggressively because we have ancillary staff to watch vital signs. I had no choice here as she refused admission. I had to go slow in pharmacotherapy as I had to treat her as outpatient.

Suma came to see me as per the scheduled appointment. She was more comfortable and allowed me to talk with the door closed. That morning she had asked her mother for coffee and drank. She had breakfast also. She didn't even say the food was poisoned. She continued that devils were after her to kill her. She went on talking for about half an hour. I didn't say anything. I just heard whatever she said. I increased her antipsychotic medicine and sent her home.

In the next two visits she reported that she was better. She said that the devils were bothering her, but she was not so much scared. This was definitely an improvement. I had to increase her medicine because she was not alright yet. I also discussed with her fear about devils. I asked her if she really believed the existence of the devils. She was not sure. If the devil was so strong why the devil didn't harm her that long? I also asked her if she had seen the devil. She denied having seen a devil. If that was the case then why she believed it? I also raised a point whether it could be her suspicion and fear. She denied it mildly. We could see even her denial was milder than before. These were the signs of improvement in her. I had to increase her medicine. She began to sleep well. Her condition improved. Her behavior became almost normal. Her fear about devils decreased, but didn't go completely. I continued to see her for about a year (initially once a week and gradually decreased to once in 3 months). She was alright at the end of one year. It is not uncommon in our society to discontinue follow up when once they are better, but she followed.

Everybody talks of the devil. Has anyone seen it? Everyone has good and bad natures in him. We attribute all good things to god and bad things to devil. Parents try to impart only good things to children and do not tolerate even a small bad thing. The child incorporates these strong feelings and tries to be completely good. He will have difficulty in accepting even a small bad thing in him. The reality is no one is perfect; even then one will not be able to accept even a small bad thing in himself. When the circumstances arise pointing towards his own bad aspect he cannot take it. If he blames the devil for those bad things it spares him from blaming himself. It is more acceptable to say the devil made him do it.

Her diagnosis is Schizophrenia. In this illness patients usually talk about being poisoned, some one or the devil trying to kill him, may hear voices, etc. These are called as delusions and hallucinations. One of the characteristics of this illness is variability. The patient may appear quite normal some time and at another time he may be very abnormal. Usually people will be misled when the patient is behaving normal at times. The incidence of this illness is about 1% in life time. Serotonin, a biochemical is found to be abnormally high in this illness. There are researches indicating some changes in the temporal lobe of the brain. A lot more research is going on in this.

If Suma didn't have treatment, what could have happened? It is a big question. I would like to report another case of the outcome in delaying. A 42 years old man was a teacher. He had one son. The problems began about 4 months ago. For about 6 to 7 days he was telling a few people were trying to kill him. His relatives would bring those people to him and make them tell him they were not at all trying to kill him. He would be alright for a while and then he would accuse some other people were trying to kill him. The relatives brought those people and made them assure him that they were not trying to kill him. He would be alright again for a while and would shift his accusation to someone else. This went on again and again and finally all got fed up. His father called me and said they wanted an emergency appointment for the next day and I obliged. He was brought to my clinic next day. He was brought on a stretcher. He was not moving any of the four limbs. I came to know that he was locked up in a room because he was violent. In the middle of the night they heard a very loud sound from his room. They were even afraid to open the door till the morning. In the morning they collected some neighbors and opened the door and he was lying on the floor. He had banged his head against the wall and had fallen on the floor. In my examination I learnt that he had damaged his spinal cord and couldn't even move his limbs. I immediately told them to take him to a big neurosurgery unit. He was taken there and neurosurgeons could not do anything because the spinal cord was badly damaged. They had to watch him succumb to death. This case is reported more in another chapter.

A long back if a person had Schizophrenia it was considered his quality of life was gone forever. The science has advanced tremendously. The psychopharmacotherapy has made a lot of progress. I would like to convey to my readers because of this advance in psychopharmacotherapy a lot of patients have gotten better and many chronic treatment hospitals have been closing down in USA. If a Schizophrenic takes treatment properly, he can lead almost normal life.

Obsessive Compulsive Disorder

Kalpana, aged 30 years was brought to me for heaviness of the head. She was accompanied by her husband and a cousin. After listening to her husband and cousin I sent them out and talked to Kalpana alone. Usually patients would not like to disclose problems in front of even their own people. It is also our ethics and duty to protect confidentiality of patient's problem. She had not disclosed all of her problems to even her husband. She was afraid that her cousin might label her as mad. She came with her cousin because her cousin knew me.

After sending her husband and cousin the first thing I witnessed was her crying. She cried for a while. I encouraged her to cry and talk only after she became comfortable. She felt sorry for crying and said she couldn't control herself. There is nothing wrong in crying. Crying is a normal emotional feeling. Feelings should not be suppressed and in fact should be expressed. Usually people do not like the sight of a person crying and they try to stop the person from crying. This is wrong. When once a person cries enough he will feel better. Instead of stopping patient from crying we should find out the reason behind it. Kalpana had treatment from many doctors and said this was her last try and she would end her life if it failed. She had heaviness of the head and stiffness in the jaw. Sometimes it was very difficult to even open her jaw. All the doctors told her that she had no physical illness. She was of the opinion that if there was no physical illness why she had this problem? She came to the conclusion that if it was not physical it must be psychological. Very few people have this much awareness about mental illness.

Kalpana's problems were of 2 years duration and had worsened for two months. She was thinking too much and was irritable. She became over concerned about cleanliness. She was feeling not clean enough even after taking bath. She started taking bath in the morning as well as at night and even then she was not feeling clean. Some days she would take bath in the afternoon also. When her husband and children came home they had to wash their feet outside and then only they were supposed to enter the house. If they ever came inside without washing their feet she would clean the whole house with water. She had to even wash walls, vessels, cans, etc. Then only she would be satisfied. Gradually her cleaning and bathing problems increased and she found it difficult to clean the whole house frequently and her husband had to help her. When her maid cleaned the vessels she had to clean them again. She would wait till the maid went home to clean the vessels again. She was afraid the maid would notice her cleaning of the vessels and tell others. Because of this fear of the maid revealing it to others she removed her from work. If her children put hand in their mouth she would just carry them to bath room and bathe them even with clothes on for fear they might touch other things. Otherwise she couldn't relax. She felt bad that she was giving so much trouble to her family. She said that she had been hell to her husband and children. She said "doctor kill me I am giving so much trouble to my husband and children". I consoled her by saying there is a cure for everything and she should not get discouraged so fast.

Even though she was from another town she came for the scheduled appointments properly. I had to see her for a total of 15 psychotherapy sessions over a period of 23 months. Initially it was once a week and gradually it was reduced to once in 2 months depending on the necessity. In psychotherapy the patient should tell what all came to his mind without any reservation. We call this as free association. Patient might talk so many things at different times, we have to keep all of them in mind and see if it made some sense when all of them put together. It is just like arranging all jumbled up pieces of the puzzle into a picture. In psychotherapy we have to put all pieces of information elicited at different times and try to make sense out of them.

Kalpana didn't like her problem of excessive cleanliness. In spite of that she could not control. This is exactly characteristic of obsessions and compulsions. They cannot stop it even though they don't like it and know it is wrong. What is causing her to do this against her own will? This is exactly her unconscious part of the mind. Her unconscious mind to compel her to do these obsessions and compulsions there must be a strong reason for it. I got some idea about it in the following visits. Her first four visits were full of crying. This was not uncommon in my experience. I had to wait for her to become comfortable. She had to develop confidence in me also. In her 5th session some important matter was revealed. When she was about 10 years old she was abused sexually by a cousin brother of around 17 years. She was not even aware what was happening. She didn't even know it was wrong. When she realized that, she felt that her body had become impure. She didn't want to marry because she didn't want to offer her impure body to her husband. In our society virginity is adored and expected. A lady who has lost her virginity is considered as impure. She told her parents that she didn't want to marry without disclosing the reason. She couldn't bring herself to tell parents the real reason for her refusal. Her parents didn't approve of her rejection for the marriage, because it would make it difficult for them to find alliances for her younger sisters. This is a common happening in our society. In our society it is a practice to arrange marriage of elder daughter first; if it is not followed it may pose difficulty in getting of her younger sisters married. She was helpless and gave consent to the marriage. After marriage she told this to her husband. He asked what exactly happened between the two. There was only touching each other's private parts. Her husband was broad minded and said that in young children do such things innocently and told her not to be worried about it.

She revealed that she had wished for brother in law's death. She would feel very bad about it. She would gently hit her cheeks and said to herself "quit, quit". Then she would feel better feeling that the sin was aborted. This was her undoing for having bad wishes of death on her brother in law. She cried saying why she got such bad thoughts. The same topic came up again and again in the subsequent visits. After she ventilated her feelings like this she felt better. This ventilating process is called as catharsis. She continued to feel better but her cleanliness problem continued. Kalpana's father was a very angry man and mother was a very mild mannered lady. She said that she had inherited her father's anger. Kalpana's husband was opposite of her in his angry nature. He would always have a smiling face. She felt because of his mild manneredness their family was facing some problems. Her father in law had left a lot of property on his death. Her husband's elder brothers took away most of it. The father in law had a good business and this elder brother of her husband took away that business and sent her husband out of the house. Her husband got one small portion in the house and loans of her father in law. Kalpana told her husband to talk to his elder brother for a proper share in the property and he scolded her and told her to keep quiet. He told her that he had not compromised in providing well for her in life and she should not worry about it.

Kalpana came with obsessions and compulsions of dirt and cleanliness. She had mentioned about her sexual act with her cousin. She felt spoiled by her sexual acts and was serving an impure body to her husband and felt guilty. She had also mentioned about death wishes on her brother in law. I began to think all these might be related in some way. Sometimes we may be doing opposite of what we think. This is called reaction formation. We can feel dirty on the one hand and clean on another other part. She was trying to wash her internal feeling of dirtiness by washing outer surface of the body. Kalpana said it was possible and there might be connection between the two, but difficult to believe.

Kalpana began to feel better. Gradually her obsessions and compulsions reduced. Initially she was free from these for some time and later was free for even 6 days a week. Ultimately she was completely alright. Any illness reduces only gradually. Then she had some relapses. She was even able to pin point the circumstances that triggered the relapse. Once she had the thoughts of her past sexual incidence and had a relapse. It was pointed out that she was not aware of the difference between adult sexuality and child sexuality. First of all as a child she was ignorant of what was happening and didn't know it was not normal. The older boy should have known it better. She realized it was bad at a later age. I had to explain that it was not an adult sexuality. There was a question on what was child sexuality. The children do indulge in touching private parts as a curiosity. That's how they learn the difference between a boy and a girl. This establishes sexual identification and orientation. She was feeling guilty because sex is a taboo in our societal values. I ascertained from her that impurity meant losing her virginity. I pointed out to her that she was not at all impure as she had not lost her virginity. She began to come to terms with it.

She was angry on her brother in law because she felt cheated about property. We all have murderous thoughts when we are angry. If entertaining murderous thoughts is a criterion to label a person as murderer then most of us will be murderers. Thoughts and actions are different. Mind should be free to think anything and everything, however bad it is. Our controls should be on our actions. If we try to suppress our bad thoughts they may find expression in action like killing. Kalpana began to accept her death wishes were very normal. Her obsessions and compulsions disappeared and she began to feel that she was normal like any other person. Her heaviness of the head and stiffness of the jaw cleared.

The diagnosis here is obsessive compulsive neurosis. The patient gets thoughts and indulges in actions repeatedly against his will. One patient had thoughts of throwing slippers on god. Another patient had thoughts of why a chair should have 4 legs and why not three legs?. One patient began feeling dirty even after a good bath. She used to get doubts whether she took a bath or not. She began writing on the calendar "GS' (good shower). That didn't satisfy her completely and doubted whether it was good shower or very good shower and she began writing on the calendar "PGS"(pretty good shower), That also didn't satisfy her and she began doubting whether she wrote it on that day or entered it wrongly on another date. In this illness if he clears one doubt another doubt will arise. This illness can be cured but takes a long time. One should not be pessimistic about outcome in mental illness.

Psychodynamics

Her external preoccupation with dirt was related to her internal feeling of dirt. This again was related to her sexual experiences and guilt associated with them. She was trying to wash her internal guilt with washing externally on the body. The guilt found expression unconsciously on to the surface of the body in terms of dirt. If one cleans some place other than where it is dirty, how the real dirt will go? This was happening in her and no amount of cleaning was enough. Compulsion to wash or bathe is also called as Ablutomania,

She had guilt about death wishes on her brother in law. Her husband was cheated out of a fair portion of his father's property.

This generated anger in her. This in turn became death wishes on the brother in law.

Sexual incidence   Body

↓   ↑ → Guilty → Wash → not satisfied → wash & wash

Dirty →   Dirty

                                                    ↓

                                              Frustration

Psychotherapy

The very first thing done was to deal with her loosing hope about the outcome of her illness. She felt guilty for causing trouble to her family by her excessive cleanliness. She was told that she was not doing deliberately and we had to understand why it was happening beyond her control. She was made aware of existence of conscious and unconscious minds and their effect on the body. Her sexual incidence and the guilt associated were dealt. Her feeling of the sexual act was dirty and sinful was discussed. She was made to realize that it was innocent children sexuality and not adult sexuality. The relation between the two dirts (sexual and outside dirt) was understood by her. She was free from heaviness of the head and stiffness of the jaw.

Her death wishes on her brother in law were related to that her husband was cheated out of fair share in ancestral property. The anger was finding expression in a passive manner (opposite to the aggressive act of killing) ie, wish for his death. All these realizations resolved the conflict between the two parts of the mind and resulted in mental harmony. Her preoccupation on dirt and washing cleared.

Attacks of Pulling Sensation

There is a lot of ignorance about mental illness. Any pain felt in the body ought to be physical is the opinion of most of the people. Psychological means it is either a lie or it is imaginary is the concept prevailing amongst public. More than 50% of all real physical symptoms are deep rooted in mind. Our conscious and unconscious minds can act through brain to cause real physical symptoms like pain etc in any part of the body. As described in a different chapter whenever there is conflict between the different parts of the mind there is generation of anxiety. Our three parts of the mind can be compared to a court. In a court there is a complainant and a defendant. The judge gives a judgment. If the judge is weak what a chaos it causes. If our ego is weak it causes chaos. This chaos is nothing, but mental turmoil leads to all types of problems. Usually an individual with well-developed ego resolves conflicts after a reasonable time. Sometimes thonflicts are so strong, and ego is not strong enough, it results in a chaotic situation and make him indecisive. Prolonged conflict with indecisiveness leads to problems. Our brain doesn't decide anything, it is our mind that decides and sends instructions through the brain. Brain is like a faithful servant of our mind. If the conflict is not resolved a confused mind sends confused messages to brain and it results in a disturbed function in the body.

When I was with a group of friends there was a casual discussion on pulling sensation of the body. The opinion of all was it was a physical problem, not even one mentioned it could be psychological. I opened the Pandora by saying pulling sensation can be pychological

Attacks of Pulling Sensation

also. It raised a lot of commotion. Some friends agreed and most of them disagreed. Our meeting ended that way. One friend called me the next day and asked me if I could help some one that he knew. He told me that they were desperate.

He sent the patient to my clinic. Rama, a 14 yrs old girl was accompanied by mother. Rama had pulling attacks with pain on her waist. Several doctors declared that she was physically alright, but her agony continued. She was taken to doctors of alternative types of medicines. She consulted even black magic and curse removal specialists, etc. This is not unusual in our society. Almost all of our patients will have undergone all types of treatment before coming to a psychiatrist. Her family was fed up of Rama's problem. It had a large financial drain on the family. Her father was a schoolteacher with a limited income. The parents had lost hope. At this stage my friend suggested my name. It came as a silver lining in a dark cloud. She was not taken to any psychiatrist, because it never occurred to them and nobody had suggested.

Rama came with clean clothes. She had Kunkum (red powder dot on the forehead worn usually by hindus) on her forehead. She was well groomed. Her actions revealed that she was a very active girl. She was well groomed. The pulling attacks with pain began on the waist while taking bath 2 years ago and worsened in the last 3 months. It was not continuous but came in attacks. She was getting attacks about 20 times a week. It was intense pain with cramps. She kept describing them as attacks. During the attacks sometimes she just stared blindly for a few seconds. Some other times she would spit saliva on her hand and smeared on her face. After the attack she would go to sleep for about 10 minutes. When she had attacks, she was observed to be in a kind of fear. She had records of various doctors ruling out any physical problem. These kinds of attacks can be due to a kind of seizures (epilepsy) also. A mere physical examination doesn't reveal any defect in a seizure individual. In a seizure individual hyperventilation induces real epilepsy. I subjected her to this test. I asked her to continue taking deep breaths for 6 minutes. It didn't induce any attacks. If it is seizures of central nervous system problem, hyperventilation for even 2 to 3 minutes will induce an attack. The thematic apperception test revealed that she was a very angry person and she wanted to be number one in everything. She was advised to see me for psychotherapy sessions.

One week later her mother brought her and said that her illness had worsened and cried. I had to comfort her by saying Rama's problem of 2 years could not be solved in one or two weeks and she had to be treated for a long time. Besides this ups and downs is natures making. All illnesses go through ups and downs. Her mother seemed to understand this and I sent her out and talked to Rama. I tried to find out from Rama if she had any disturbances in her mind and what circumstances had led to attacks in that week. She denied any upsetting incidents. I delved what all she did in that week. I learnt that one day she wanted to go to a party with her friends and mother refused permission because Rama might get an attack and it might become public and all might label as mad. Her problem becoming public might cause difficulty in her marriage chances in the future. Following mother's denying the permission she had 3 attacks. At that time her mother even felt guilty that she didn't allow her to go and even thought attacks might have not happened if she had permitted her to go.

Treatment continued with weekly therapy sessions. Another time Rama asked her father money to buy something. Her father refused to give money saying it was not necessary. Following this she had an attack. At this stage I had to reassure her mother that her illness was not serious one and not to be afraid so much. I also suggested her to downplay the reactions whenever Rama had attacks. A psychiatrist has to deal with others also, whenever necessary. Rama's frustration and dejection continued. She asked me to give her something to die. She said she was not needed by anybody. Her parents were so much concerned and asked her why she felt like not needed by anybody. She admitted that they loved her. She said that her parents were more worried about her problem of becoming known to others. For my question of whether it was wrong on the part of her parents to feel that way, she had no response. I asked her whether it was alright for her, if it became public. She also said that she didn't want it to be public. At this stage she felt sorry for being angry on her parents for this reason. In one week, she had 20 attacks and out of them we had a definite indication in 5 attacks to feel the attacks occurred whenever she was upset. I have not described the circumstances in which other attacks happened, which occurred in similar circumstances also. I pointed out to Rama in details how her attacks were related to getting upset about something or the other.

Her father's financial position was not very good as mentioned earlier. She was to see me for a session one day and she asked her father for money. Her father refused to give her money without even finding out what for she wanted. She gathered all small changes that she had with her and came. I was very happy about it as it showed her strong motivation to get better. She didn't have an attack also, which was a very positive development. I told her that she should not get upset whenever she was denied of something. She should try to see if she could achieve it in some other way like this time, if it is so important and reasonable. I even appreciated for her very mature and appropriate behavior at that stage.

In the following sessions many things became apparent. Rama hated to hear "no" from anyone and for anything. When denied something she would get extremely disturbed. In the 5 (only circumstances of 2 attacks have been described) attacks that she had were related for denial of something. She reluctantly agreed. As stated above she wanted to be first always. She should be first for her parents love also. In the past she had complained that parents loved and cared more for her sister than her. I raised the issue if parents loved her siblings did it meant that parents loved her less? Human being is capable of loving many people at the same time, where is the question of more or less love? Rama loved both of her parents and she couldn't even say whom she loved more. She agreed for this and even felt bad for her silly behavior (she described it like this). I consoled her by saying that she was young and there was a lot to learn in life yet. Her reaction was not uncommon at all. At this stage she recalled that she had some attacks whenever she felt parents showed love towards her siblings.

She was very angry natured and was very angry when her parents were unable to satisfy her wants. Her father was a middle class person with financially limited resources. He had to manage the family within his means. I asked Rama did she know anyone who got what all one wanted. This is the fact of life. All of us get only some things and not all. This is the truth of life. We should learn to be happy for what we get and accept with bitterness for what we don't get. She in fact thanked me for opening her knowledge about life. She was also a part of the family and should understand the difficulties of running the family. Her demands should be affordable for the family. She agreed. It was pointed out to her that she was unknowingly trying to get what she wanted through illness. It was also a fact that parents have to treat children differently for various reasons like age, circumstances, illness, etc,etc eg: Two years elder sister's needs may be different than that of an younger sister. It is not discrimination, but the needs are different at different ages. If a sibling is not well, he requires more care at that time. These are facts of life. She seemed to take all these things in good spirit. Rama's illness served the purpose of demanding more attention of parents.

I was quite well aware of Rama"s illness at this stage. Our treatment had a positive effect. Her attacks had reduced from 20 per week to about 5 per week but had not stopped. In spite of so much therapy her problem was not cured. Here we must understand that her body and mind were adapted to the illness. Our body and mind will get adapted to good or bad things unknowingly. This we call as conditioning. I decided to subject her to deconditioning therapy. I subjected her to SEDAC treatment. In this I asked her to remember her attacks and passed a small current to her temples through a treatment machine. This is not the same as Shock treatment (electro convulsive therapy). Sedac is given in a conscious state and anesthesia is not given. The current is just enough to make the patient unpleasant while she thought of attacks. Gradually mind starts associating attacks with the unpleasant stimulus and makes it undesirable. This called deconditioning therapy. This is based on Pavlov's conditioning.

Pavlov demonstrated like this. He proposed that a neutral stimulus can be made to be a positive stimulus. He demonstrated in dog. He rang the bell and measured the acidity in the dog, there was no increase in the stomach acidity. Next he rang the bell and kept food in front, there was increase in acidity. After repeatedly doing like that he just rang the bell without keeping food in front, still there was increase in acidity. Here neutral stimulus became a positive stimulus. This he labeled it as conditioning response. In Sedac the same principle is used for deconditioning.

Pavlov's conditioning theory: -

He demonstrated on dog.

1. Rang the bell → no increase in acidity
2. Rang the bell + food → increase in acidity

   After a few times

3. Rang the bell → increase in acidity

A neutral stimulus (bell) had become a positive stimulus.

After a few Sedac treatments Rama was free of attacks. The question here is whether Rama was faking the problem? In fact her parents had raised this question to me. She was definitely not faking. A faking person will not have strain on his face. He will not bother about his illness and even doesn't participate in treatment properly. He will not do anything to deprive him of what he enjoys to do. His attacks happen in different circumstances at different times.

Then why she had this problem? Her instinctual drive was narcistic (selfish and wanted more love from the parents). Her material needs were not met by parents for financial constraints. This was the desire of her unconscious mind. However, her conscious mind hated it. The resulting conflict was unresolved. It resulted in her attacks. Her ego (partly not matured enough, in a 14 yrs old girl) was not able to solve. Being aware of the problem stopped her unconscious mind from giving troubles. Her longing to be first and not understanding of the reality like her parent's financial position, etc helped her. She was completely alright even after one month. In the next 3 months I discontinued her medicines gradually. Believe it ore not in our next meeting with group of friends my friend, who sent Rama was the first to say physical symptoms can be a manifestation of deep-rooted psychological problems. Here the question arises why her problem was not solved by just giving sedac treatment alone. Sedac treatment is a symptomatic treatment. If only sedac treatment was given her problem would have relapsed after some time, because the root cause of the problem was not treated. Psychodynamic psychotherapy was also carried out to remove the root cause of the problem.

Living In The Past

A 62 years old person, Prasad came to me accompanied by his wife and his brother. He had sleep difficulty for 4 years and it was worse in the last 20 days. He said he had not slept at all for those 20 days. He felt tired and got fed up about this problem. He even preferred death than this agony. His wife told him not to talk of death. His wife denied any problem between them and said he was a good husband. She was worried about his problem. I sent wife and brother outside to talk to Prasad alone.

He was living in his own house and had own business. He owned the building in which he was carrying out his business. He had one daughter married and settled in USA. The daughter and son in law got along very well and there were no worries about them. He had a wholesale business of selling paper. The business was dull, because of intense competition. It was an ancestral business and he was managing along with his brother. He also had money lending as side business. He would give loans for a few well-known people for a much higher interest than banks. It was a joint family and his brother's family shared the same house. They got along well. His wife and his brother's wife got along very well. His brother had two daughters who were married and settled well with their own families. The mental status examination revealed minor depression and some anxiety, otherwise alright. The physical examination was alright. There was no history of treatment for any physical problem. I prescribed a tranquilizer and an antidepressant with a suggestion to come for psychotherapy sessions.

He had an ancestral property in his native town. It was vacant. He had not given it for rent. Many times, he had to go and take care of repairs, etc. it was an old house and it needed repairs often. He got fed up in maintaining that house. Both he and his brother decided to sell. He sold the house 4 years ago. He felt bad about that decision of selling the house, where as his brother didn't feel bad like him. He felt bad If he had kept it he would have gotten a lot better price.

He missed his daughter. He was very close to her. She was a software engineer and had a very well- paying job. He always wanted to arrange for her marriage to a person living nearby his house so that he could see her quite often. He was feeling that he had made a mistake in arranging for her marriage with a person settled in USA. He didn't know what had happened to him at the time of arranging for the marriage. He said it was a blunder. His daughter was very happy with her husband. His son in law was a good person. Realizing his agony his son in law offered tickets for them to visit them in USA. Prasad had self-pride and didn't want to accept it and he couldn't afford with his own money to visit them frequently. He had already visited them once with his own expenditure. He was quite happy to see the good relationship of his daughter and son in law. His agony was in case he wanted to see his daughter or if there was an emergency, he could not bear the expenditure of going to see her. Realizing this his son in law offered to send his daughter whenever he wanted to see her. This was not satisfying him.

There were two factors here, he was a worrying type of a person and was living in the past. He felt bad for his past decisions. Prasad said his business was dull, because of severe competition. Before his business was good, hence he didn't think of investing his money in real estate. His friends suggested him in the past to invest in real estate and he did not heed for it. His friends who invested in real estate had made more money. There were good real estate offers and he thought he was better with money lending at that time. He never thought the real estate would appreciate better than money lending. He cursed himself saying he was stupid.

He had said that he didn't sleep for 20 days. This was impossible. People become psychotic with even one week of not having full sleep. This is well established in sleep laboratories. In the laboratory they have taken people who claimed of not having sleep at all for days together and found out they had sleep and just it was not registered in the mind. This was established through EEG(Electro encephalogram). When a person sleeps it shows sleep spindles. People worry too much for not getting sleep. The more we try, the less we will be successful in getting sleep. Our body will take necessary required sleep. We should not try to meddle with it.

He accepted he was a worrying type of person. With whatever he had he could live comfortably but was worried if he had to make USA trips it would be financially straining. If he had more money he would have not worried about going to USA. He was worrying in anticipation of some emergency for which he might have to go USA. This showed his pessimism and insecurity. If we worry too much of uncertain future, we will have a whole world of worriers. When everything is going well, we should learn to enjoy. Who knows the future may be good also. When a person loses hope everything looks bleak. We should give more importance to the present with a less importance to the future and least importance to the past. We shouldn't let go the present happiness. The present is in front of us and we should enjoy. Future is important, because what we do today will have some foundation for the future. The past is important to learn from our past mistakes and to correct the future mistakes. Looking at the past should not be for repenting about the past mistakes. Prasad was repenting for not investing in real estate, selling the ancestral property and arranging marriage for his daughter with a person settled abroad.

Psychodynamics

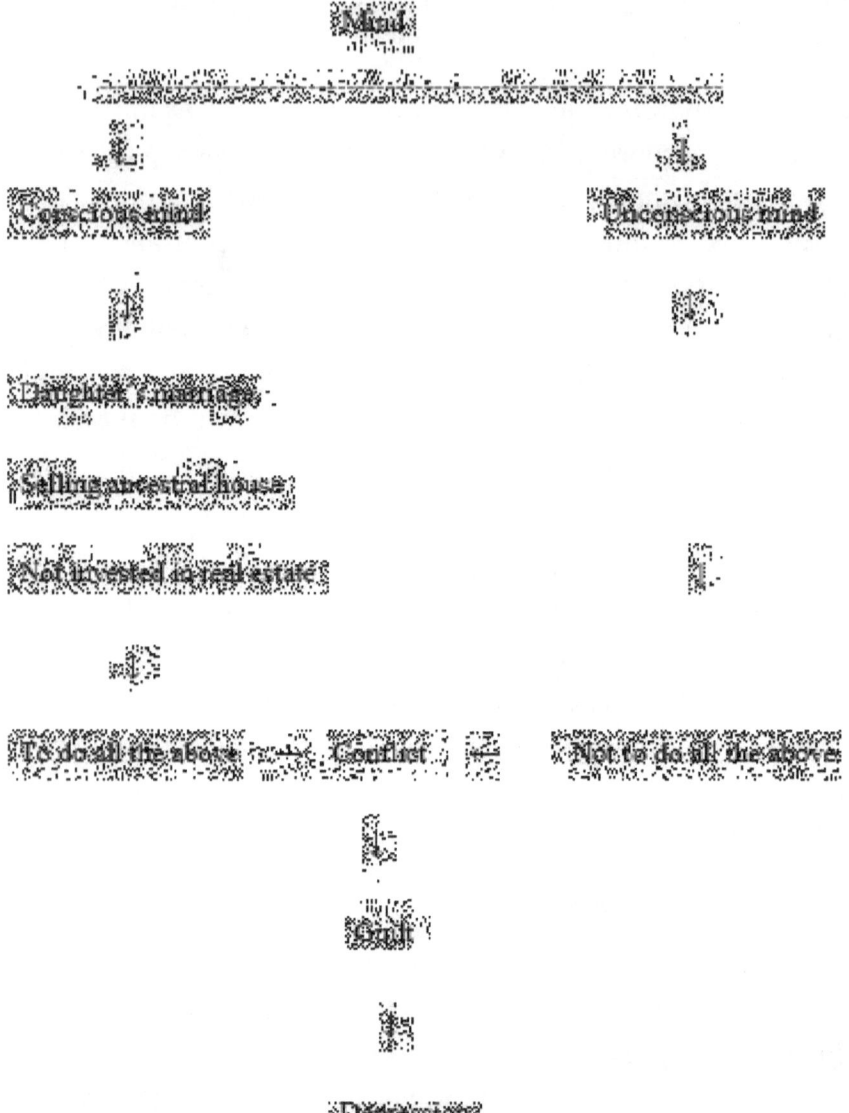

Prasad felt guilty for about three matters as mentioned above. The unconscious mind never accepted completely to carry out all of them. This guilt unconsciously made him live in the past. His unconscious mind continued to torment him for the past wrong doings as per himself. There was no way to go back to the past and rectify it and he wouldn't accept them also. The resulting conflict led to the depression.

Psychotherapy

He was allowed to ventilate his so-called wrongdoings. It was brought to his notice that it had happened in the past. He was pointed out that he was living in the past rather than in present. One should try to forget the past and live in the present. It was pointed out that no one could undo the past. He should have been contented that his daughter was well settled, and he had enough to live for the present and future.

I raised a point to tell me in case he rejected the marriage proposal of his daughter, how he would have felt. He could not answer that. Knowing him I said that probably he would have felt guilty for rejecting a good proposal. He was one of many such people who do one thing then feel sorry for doing it. If he didn't do it, he would have felt sorry for not doing. Either way he would feel sorry. It is their mental makeup (felt sorry). Some people are good in feeling sorry later for not deciding for the other alternative.

Prasad accepted psychotherapy revelations. He said he would begin to live in the present. There were some other things that needed to be addressed. He was just sitting at home and brooding. I told him to resume meeting his friends and his walking. I asked him to take trips. He could also cultivate some hobbies. He decided to attend some religious discourses. The therapy was terminated. Prasad was a perfectionist. He wanted the best of everything. He was not tolerating even a small mistake. He was the type who would make decisions and then repent. It took 9 psychotherapy sessions to make him realize his problem.

Greed

Anand was a 52 years old male came to me with complaints of poor sleep for 1.5 years. He was not getting good sleep. He had a wife with a son and a daughter. It was a nuclear family. He had a business of money lending. He lent money to about 30 well known and rich businesspeople. Sometimes he got headaches, chest discomfort, back ache, etc. He was worried it might be heart attack, stroke, etc. He had been to his family physician many times and each time the physician gave a verdict that Anand had no physical illness. He was taking about 8 medications per day. He was fed up of physical symptoms and taking so many medications. Anand felt if he had no physical illness, why he should take so many medicines. The physician said it was for treating the symptoms.

My psychiatric evaluation revealed that he had some anxiety and depression. He said that he had difficulty in falling asleep and would wake up three to four times in the night. When he woke up, he needed more time to fall asleep again. In the morning he would wake up being not satisfied of having enough sleep. Just like all of us differ in our personality characteristics, our sleep pattern also varies. Some people can sleep and get up any time. Some people wake up several times and still may have enough sleep. Some people must sleep and get up at a certain time only. Most of the people sleep around 7 hours per day. We know of people sleeping only 3 to 4 hours without any loss of function. A good example is big national leaders, who have to face all very big issues with only 3to 4 hours of sleep. I tried to ascertain whether his problem of sleep was his natural pattern, or it was not normal. He had no sleep problem 1.5 years ago. If it was his natural pattern, perhaps he would have not come to me at all. Satisfaction of sleep is the criteria for a person of having enough sleep. He was not satisfied with his sleep. This indicated that he had a problem of sleep.

Then the next question in my mind was why he had sleep problem for 1.5 years. He couldn't answer for this. Here the important thing was both patient and I were not aware of the problem. Only the problem was in the unconscious mind and I had to get it out. I had to give him some antidepressants and antianxiety agents for temporary relief. The psychotherapy sessions continued. A couple of sessions continued without accomplishing much. I had to be patient and yet probing. One time he said that he was fed up of income tax people. He said he was afraid of them. He didn't reveal further about it in that session. In a later session he said that his business involved accumulation of black money. He admitted because of this he was afraid. Gradually all these and further information came out as pieces of information. Ultimately, I learnt that he had hoarded a lot of black money and he was afraid of IT (income tax) raid. If it happened, he would lose all the money and had to undergo punishment also. In the day time he was afraid of IT raid and at night he was afraid of antisocial elements would break in and it might be dangerous to life also. As a result, he was afraid the whole day and night and wouldn't get sleep at night. He agreed that he shouldn't have resorted to dodging taxes and there was no way of undoing of the past. I was also not sure what I could do at that stage of treatment. At that stage all I could do was to give him symptomatic treatment.

Anand was a miserly person. He was restricting the family to spend only for the necessities. Even his wife had expressed why it was necessary to lead such a frugal life, when he had so much money. He never changed. He believed one should earn and save as much as possible. He was also of the opinion that it was his hard-earned money and why he should pay taxes to the government. He said in this corrupt world his taxes would be embezzled by politicians. He thought that dodging taxes was a socially accepted matter, and everybody was doing it. He didn't feel guilty about it.

He was living a frugal life as described above. It was in newspapers that government began cracking down on black money holders. Some people's black money was confiscated, and they were put in prison. This worried him. He thought if that were to happen to him what he would do. He was scared that he would lose all his money and might end up in prison. Also, there was an incident of theft and killing of a person for money kept in the house. This again aggravated his anxiety. He began to worry and lost sleep. These incidents happened 1.5 years prior to his symptoms.

At this stage I knew about what exactly the problem was. The solution was not there, even though the root cause of the problem was already known. The offence of not declaring his income properly had been done. At that stage a declaration would involve losing most of his money and severe punishment. I told him at that time only thing that was possible to give him some relief by medicines only. He was fed up of taking medicines and there was no other solution. He was afraid that he might have to go on like this for ever of taking medicines. He had lost hope. I advised him never to lose hope and he might get a chance. He was pessimistic and I kept telling him not to lose hopes and be optimistic. This continued for about 10 months.

Luck doesn't strike always; it strikes sometimes only. We must make use of it by grabbing it when it strikes. For his luck suddenly the government announced a policy for the black money holders. There was an announcement that anyone can declare his black money by paying 30% tax and there would not be any penalty. Anand came to me with that newspaper cutting. I asked him what he was going to do. He didn't want to part with 30% of his money. He was silent when I asked him what might happen if he didn't use this opportunity. He said that he might have to continue to suffer. If this state continued, he might even end up in severe illnesses, like acidity, blood pressure, heart attack, etc. He asked me what he should do. I told him that I could not decide this, and it was his decision only. He had only two options at that stage, either to declare or to continue to suffer like that. He stated that he was worried about losing 30% of his money. He had to decide between health and money. If he decided to declare he would retain 70% of money. Being a very calculative man, I asked him how much he would get if he invested it in fixed deposit for five years. He said that he might get about 50 to 60% more. I also asked him how much his black money will be if he kept it at home for five years. He said it would remain the same. At that stage he realized that he was better off after five to ten years if he declared the black money. Also, he will have good sleep and would not have fears of IT or thieves. His health would be better also.

He decided to go ahead with the declaration. I suggested him to talk to his auditor and decide. Later Anand told me his auditor endorsed it and he was going to declare. Amazingly he had a very good relief from his symptoms when once he made the decision. He became completely alright after he declared it officially. Readers might wonder what I was doing talking about accounts, he realized that he was better in all respects by declaring to the government. I firmly believe that my goal was to relieve my patient of his problem. There is nothing wrong in talking about account matters, if it were the cause of his illness. His treatment prolonged because there was no solution available for several months.

Selfishness and greed are the characteristics of ID (child instinctual part). His superego (parent part) had accepted with dodging taxes because it was a socially accepted crime. A lot of people were doing it and it was very common. His ego (adult part) accepted it and he was functioning without any problems (homeostasis). The IT raids and thefts altered the homeostasis. Because of the fear of being caught superego became harder. The ego was helpless as there was no solution to the problem. For several months his suffering continued. The result of it was insomnia, depression, anxiety, etc. When the government announced a scheme for the black money holders the ego had an option. Yet he was reluctant and agreed when once he came to know he would be better off in the long run by declaring. I was happy that his problem ended in a positive manner. The treatment was prolonged here because there was no solution to his problem for several months till the government announced a new scheme.

Psychodynamics

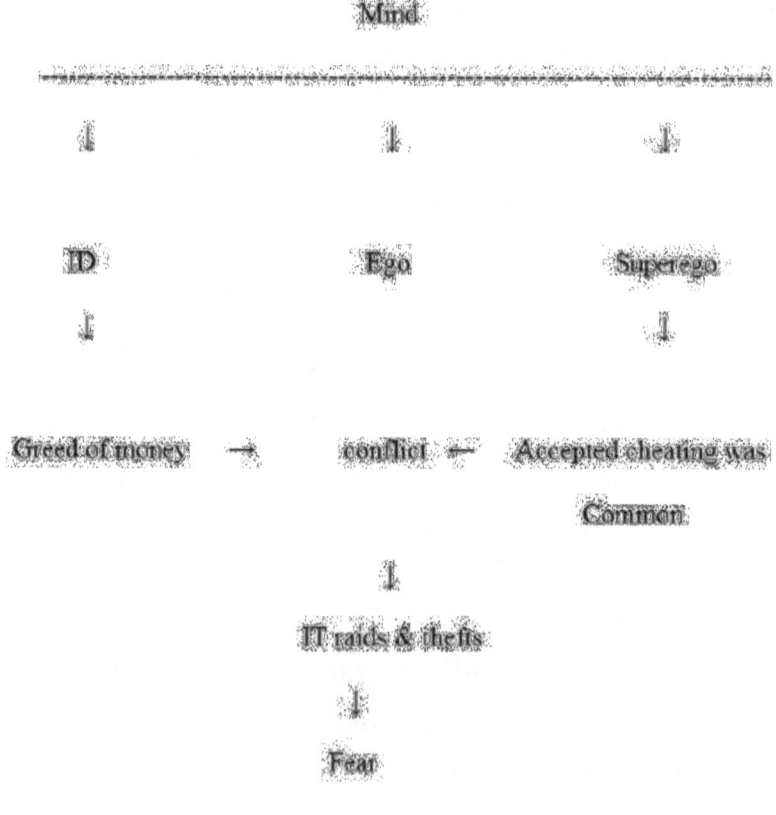

Anand was greedy about money. This is ID's instinct. The tax cheating was prevailing widely in the society. The superego, which decides right and wrong was satisfied because it was a common happening in the society. As it was alright with ID and Superego there was no conflict. He was able to function in harmony. The Income tax raids and thefts altered the homeostasis of the mind. He developed Anxiety, poor sleep and somatic symptoms.

Psychotherapy

At first there was identification of the problem. He was not able to adjust to the altered situation like IT raids and thefts. He recognized his greed for money. He was afraid of his hoarding a lot of money. He was self-centered and was of the opinion that whatever that he earned should be for him only and why the taxes had to be paid to the government.

The altered situation made him realize that he was better in the long run by declaring and paying taxes. He realized that it was affecting his health also. He realized in therapy health is even more important than money. As it was committed already and there was no way to rectify it for some time. He was losing patience and in therapy I advised him not to lose hopes. For his luck the government announced a scheme for tax dodgers. He was hesitant because he would lose 30% in taxes. In psychotherapy he learnt that he was better of by grabbing the opportunity. He also learnt that he could lead a more peaceful life by declaring. He learnt life was not just for making money and it had to be enjoyed also.

Paralysis

Lakshmi was a good example for psychological problem that can cause physical problem. Her problem is known as Hysteria in psychiatry. Once upon a time in Greece it was believed that root cause of paralysis in women was in uterus, hence the word hysteria. Hysteria may manifest as paralysis, pain in different parts of the body, convulsions, loss of touch sensation, sleep walking, loss of hearing, loss of vision, forgetfulness, etc. It can manifest as split or multiple personality also. Sometimes a real physical problem can be superimposed with hysterical problem. In such cases even the best treatment for the physical problem cannot cure the illness, unless underlying hysteria is also treated. Hysteria is not madness. People with hysteria are generally quite intelligent and it is a curable disease.

One Monday morning I reached my clinic at 10 am as usual. Usually Monday mornings are somewhat hectic, and I began seeing my patients. The receptionist called me and said that I had a call from a doctor. He was running a nursing home in Bangalore. I was a consultant in that nursing home. He asked me to see Lakshmi with paralysis. I told him that he should be calling a neurologist, instead of me. He said that she was already seen and treated by a neurologist and there was no improvement. He wanted my opinion on this.

Paralysis can happen in neurological (nervous system pathology) and in psychological problems. Before assuming it is psychological, we must rule out any neurological problem. After seeing all patients in my clinic, I drove to the nursing home. Lakshmi was a 22 years lady and looked like a village lady, but seemed to be intelligent. She talked with no interest and seemed to be preoccupied. Her hands were trembling. Her problem began about a month ago. She had menstrual problem and had a minor surgery on her uterus. Two days after the surgery she had swelling with pain on her right thigh. She underwent oil massage and applied hot fomentation on right thigh. It reduced the swelling, but pain remained. She went to a general practitioner and he gave two injections. Three days later she could not get up from the bed in the morning. She could not even move her right leg. She was admitted to a big hospital for one week with no improvement. She performed pooja and even saw a mantravadi (mantravadi supposed to cure people of their illness by chanting religious mantras). She began having heavy bleeding from her vagina and she was treated at the nursing home. She was admitted for excessive bleeding and not for paralysis.

My next task was to assess whether her paralysis was neurological or psychological. Reflexes, pain and touch sensation didn't reveal much information. She looked preoccupied and depressed. This was not enough to say it was psychological, because even a real neurological patient would be depressed. At the end of my examination I was not sure whether it was psychological. The next morning, I subjected her for Narco Examination. It is commonly known as truth serum test. A small amount of pentothal was given so that person would become half unconscious and lose conscious control of himself. Under this condition I asked her to move her right leg and she did. Meanwhile one of the nurses had told me that she had moved her right leg in the night. Both indicated that her problem was psychological.

Next day Lakshmi denied of having any worries as an answer to my question. Sometimes we must wait patiently and create a situation to make the patient comfortable to express freely. The patient also must develop confidence in the doctor. Slowly she began talking. She was married for seven years. She had studied up to PUC. Her mother died when she was only three months old. She hardly remembered anything about her mother. Her father died about two years ago. Father remarried after her mother's death. The stepmother gave a lot of trouble to her and her brothers. Once Lakshmi ate something without asking her stepmother and she chopped lakshmi's two fingertips. Lakshmi had seven elder brothers and they were very fond of her. She had no sisters. Lakshmi had faced severe problem with her step mother and if that was the problem she should have her illness soon after that. I felt that there must be some other problem also.

I saw her on third day. There was no change in her illness. I tried to find out if any incidence happened about a month earlier and I failed. Even though it was my third visit her husband had not come to see me even once. This was unusual to me. When I asked her about her husband, she broke down with inconsolable crying. She had intense crying describing about her problem with her husband. Seven years back Lakshmi was studying in college. She was quite intelligent. One of her brothers would leave her to college and pick her up after the college. One day her brother came late. It was already dark, and everybody had gone away. Only one mason was there. He took advantage of her helpless situation and raped her. Her life became bad after the incidence. Her father was still alive at that time. A police complaint was given, and the mason was put in jail. After this incidence her family began looking down upon her. They were worried about their family prestige and never thought what impact it had on Lakshmi. Father and brothers got the mason out of jail with a condition that he would marry her. They never tried to find out the feelings of Lakshmi in regard to marrying him.

After the marriage her parents and brothers were not visiting and talking to her. They barred her from coming to their home. If she wanted to meet them it had to be in a lonely place. They were afraid that someone would see them talking to her. She felt like an outcaste. They would give her money. What lakshmi wanted was some love and affection. The next day Lakshmi was better and a little cheerful. She had good sleep for the first time after the illness began. Till now her appetite was poor and she was eating as a routine. She began experiencing hunger. All these were good signs. Her paralysis remained the same.

I told Lakshmi that she had no neurological defect that could be responsible for her paralysis and it was psychological. Her immediate reaction was that she was not lying and acting. I told her that she was not faking. I explained to her about the presence of unconscious mind. Her deep-rooted feelings might be responsible for her problem. I told her that we had observed that the movement in her right leg in her sleep and in narco test. The paralysis might be serving a deep-rooted purpose.

At this point Lakshmi said that she worked as a tailor and earned around 200 rupees per month. A psychiatrist must be vigilant. The subconscious mind comes out in a matter of fact manner. Sometimes the pieces of information come out at different times and if we put them together it will give some meaning. It is like arranging a puzzle. Sometimes when we tell something the patient may tell something else, which appears as though it is an irrelevant response.

We shall go back to her response for my statement that her paralysis might be serving some deeprooted psychological purpose. She said that she earned about 200 rupees per month. It looks as though it was an irrelevant response. Apparently, she was dragging me unconsciously for something to be explored further about her work and earnings. She was not able to use tailoring machine because of her paralysis. She was not able to earn that some small amount also. Her husband would come and go at any time. When he came whatever money, she had he would take and go away.

He never contributed for house expenditure. In the beginning her father and brothers gave her money and after her father's death brothers continued monetary support. Lately her self-pride made her not to ask money from her brothers. She was maintaining with what she was getting from tailoring. After paralysis that income also stopped. What was the outcome, she would have to go hungry and die ultimately? At that point she admitted entertaining suicidal thoughts, but she was not able to carry it out, because she had a child also. Out of the meagerly earned money she would save a little and kept it secretly in her house. Husband found out the hiding place and took away that money also. She was very disturbed about it. This happened just a couple of days prior to her paralysis.

Soon after her marriage she learnt that her husband was already married, and his first wife was alive. Whenever he was angry, he would go to his first wife. Lately he was coming less frequently to Lakshmi's house. If he came, he would give a lot of troubles and even would hit her. Lakshmi tolerated all these just to keep the husband for the name sake. People give trouble to a lonely lady. During those 4 days she cried a lot talking about her problems. Everyday mostly it was a crying session. After she cried so much there was a relief and she became more comfortable. I made her sit on the bed leaving the legs down. I told her to look at her right leg and kick her left leg up and down. I told her to keep doing like that for some time. Lakshmi became more cheerful and her brothers also visited her, which also helped. Her right leg witnessed small movements. I asked her to try kicking her right leg as she was doing with her left leg. She was able to do it. Then I asked her to hold the cot and walk. The next day when I went to see her whole lot of staff and others greeted me saying Lakshmi was walking. Behind them Lakshmi came walking with a smile. Her touch sensation became normal. She was discharged with an instruction for follow up as an outpatient. During follow up I was able to convince her brothers to pay attention to her.

Psychodynamics

Marital problem

```
Family negligence
      ↓
  Depression
      ↓
  Life instinct
To live for the child  →  conflict  ←  Suicidal Thoughts
                            ↓
                        Death wish
                            ↓
                        Paralysis of leg
                            ↓
                       Not able to do tailoring
                            ↓
                       Loss of income to live
                            ↓
                       Death not able to live
                        (Passive suicide)
```

We shall look at psychodynamics in this case. She was in extreme depression following rape, marriage and being disowned by her father and brothers. Even though husband was not looking after her she was leading life with what her brothers gave and from earnings of tailoring. Later her self-pride made her to deny her brothers monetary help. Her husband would take away even small amount which she had earned. Imagine her pathetic situation. She thought of suicide and held back because of child. Here we can see the conflict between her two minds. On the one hand she wanted to die because of her pathetic condition and on the other hand she wanted to live for the sake of her child. Her life situation was getting worse and it was becoming difficult for her to live. Her unconscious mind caused paralysis. This would deprive her of meager income. The paralysis served the indirect purpose of dying. What she couldn't bring herself to do consciously was trying to achieve it unconsciously. This can be considered as passive suicide, because she thought that illness could cause death. The result of suicide or illness is same ie. death.

Psychotherapy

The first thing after ascertaining it was psychological was telling her problem was not neurological and it was definitely psychological. I got her to reveal her worries. As she spoke about her worries there was an improvement in her depression. The medicines also helped. She became aware of her wish to commit suicide and desire for living for the sake of the child. As there was no scope for improvement in her life, the unconscious mind resorted to death wish. She became aware of how her unconscious mind was trying to drag her to death unknowingly. The brothers began visiting her after I talked to them. This helped her also. I encouraged her to kick her right leg at first and then both the legs. She was given medicines for depression.

People are highly sentimental and gullible. After Lakshmi got better the information spread widely in the area. I was flooded with calls from seven patients with paralysis from that region. All were neurological paralysis. I had a hell of a time in convincing them that it was not in my specialty. Some didn't even agree with that. They even tried to bring influence and offered me more money. They thought that I was not interested in them. It was difficult for me to convince them that I could not help them.

Paranoid Delusion

A doctor is considered as god in the society. People have a lot of trust in doctors. They expect him to cure all the problems, after all he is considered as god. If his illness is not cured the doctor is cursed. Nowadays a doctor is taken to courts if the illness is not cured. A doctor is only a human being and he can do only the maximum of what a doctor can do. Often people are not ready to accept it.

Many times, an old patient will refer another patient for treatment. In that way I received a call from someone mentioning my old patient's name. He said that illness was severe and requested me for an appointment on the very next day. They came for consultation. The father said they came from about 60 kilometers away. He was brought in a taxicab as he was not in a condition to be brought in a bus. He was brought at around 11 am.

Ravi, the patient was 42 years old. He was married and had three children. He was a cloth merchant. Seven people had accompanied him, and all were very anxious. Some were even crying. Ravi's problem began 4 months ago and had become severe in last 7 days. In the beginning he started telling his wife that someone was trying to kill him. His wife ignored it and kept quiet. Sometimes later she would reassure him saying that nobody would kill him. Initially he used to be satisfied with it and used to keep quiet for a while. Gradually that kind of assurance from his wife was not enough. He didn't let his wife turn off the lights at night for fear that someone might kill him. He would cover windows with thick cloths so that no one could see inside. He would even cover up keyhole in the door to avoid people from looking inside. He feared someone was watching and would kill him at an appropriate time. When his wife couldn't handle it anymore, she brought it to the attention of others in the family.

Someone in the family began advising him that he need not worry and all of them were with him for support. They told Ravi even though he was lean built, he was quite strong enough to defend himself. Someone else told him that he was a good man, and nobody would kill a good man. Someone else said that he was a man and why he should be afraid like a woman. None seemed to work, and his fear kept increasing. Ravi began to hear voices telling" your life is finished". Ravi's fear increased. The parents thought the god was angry with them for some reason. They performed worships and homas (A fire is set up for worship. It is a ritual). They brought people to remove the evil spirit. The spiritual healers were also brought in and none gave any relief. In fact, it got worsened.

As per the suggestion of some, the father would bring the people on whom Ravi was accusing and made them assure Ravi that they were not going to kill him. This would satisfy Ravi for a while only and later he would name some others were trying to kill him. His father would bring them also to convince him and again he would blame some other people. This kept on going. Finally, they concluded that it was of no use to convince him. At that time, they happened to meet one of my old patients and he suggested them to bring him to me. They were reluctant to bring him to me for the fear that others would think that Ravi was mad.

The family had a meeting of all members in that night and finally decided to bring him to me. The father informed it was serious and requested me for an appointment on the very next day itself and I obliged. He was brought to my clinic on the next day. They reported that he was very violent in the last couple of days. They were even afraid to go near him. They locked him up in his room whole night. In the middle of that night they heard a very loud sound from his room and after that he was quiet, but they were afraid to open the door at night because of his violence. In the morning they took the help of some people and opened the door. They found him lying on the floor. He didn't even get up. They lifted him and put him in a taxi and brought him to my clinic.

Ravi greeted me with a smile. He claimed that his life was in danger as some people were trying to kill him. He also claimed that someone present in my clinic was trying to kill him. He reported hearing voices telling him his life was over. He said that his entire story was broadcasted on television. He said that previous night the voices had become intolerable and being unable to bear he banged his head against the wall and fell to the ground. He reported severe pain in the back of his neck. I looked at it and the neck were swollen. He had lost control of all the limbs. I realized that his spinal cord was broken, and I suggested him to be taken to a famous neurosurgery hospital. He required emergency surgery to see if his spinal cord could be repaired.

Neurosurgeon saw him and had a consultation with another senior neurosurgeon. Ravi's spinal cord was damaged to the extent of beyond repair. The condition was not operable at all. The family painfully had to watch Ravi succumbing to death slowly. What an agony for the family? Delay and negligence can result in a disaster.

The diagnosis here is schizophrenia. There are different types in schizophrenia. The common type is paranoid type. This usually affects young adults. What people usually call as mad is schizophrenia. Because of ignorance and stigma people label all those going to a psychiatrist as mad. Nowadays the prognosis for Schizophrenia is far better. We have a whole lot of medications available.

The biggest problem in treating a schizophrenic is the defense mechanism of denial. The patient denies of having any problem and hence refuses to see a psychiatrist and take medications. His contention is if he has no illness why he should he take medications, but all other people know that he is not normal. Another characteristic of this illness is variability. The patient fluctuates between normal and abnormal behaviors. The family gets misled by his intermittent normal behavior and delays in seeking treatment. This misled Ravi's family in seeking treatment. If he was brought one day before he could have been saved. This is a good example of negligence resulting in a disaster. Often the negligence is because of stigma and ignorance.

Uncontrolled Neck Movements

Human life is full of problems. Nobody likes problems, but everyone must face them. Life without problems is like food without spices. We don't realize problems make us more mature and face life in a better way in the future. One who has tasted bitter can enjoy the taste of sweet more. Profession is part and parcel of life. We must face challenging situations sometimes. These challenging situations are like spices in the food. When we are successful in those challenges, we will be happy. Life cannot be without challenges. I faced this in the following treatment venture.

Nagaraj, a 45 years old man was referred by a family physician. He had uncontrolled movements of his neck (head nodding) and couldn't turn his neck to the left (torticollis) for about a year. He had neck pain also. He would flex his neck and extend it uncontrollably. It was a repetitive action. His head used to nod front and back continuously. The family physician had ruled out all physical problems and then had sent him to me.

As per the patient about a year back it began with a back pain. He was given calcium injection. It relieved back pain, but it was followed by fever. As the fever began his neck turned towards right side and he couldn't move the neck to the left. Fever subsided but the neck remained turned to the right. No matter how much he tried he couldn't turn his neck to the left. Gradually neck pain and head nodding began. Nagaraj was working in another state and had consulted many specialists there with no avail. Finally, he consulted a family physician who was also his relative here and he directed him to consult me.

Nagaraj wanted a faster cure as he was offered a job in another state. He wanted to get back to join his new job. He was given two months' time to get cured and join the new job. His head nodding and torticollis was more in the evenings and whenever he was upset. He was married for 25 years and had two children. He had no problem in the family. After two years of college (intermediate of those days) he was employed in a film distributing company for twenty years. The company incurred loss and had to be closed. He had earned a good name in that company. Nagaraj was very much upset at that time. He had a good reputation as a worker and got a job in another film distributing company. He worked there for three years and was relieved from there to accommodate a owner's close relative. He became unemployed for the last one and a half years. He had received some money as parting salary and had spent half of it already. His son was studying in engineering college. Nagaraj's father was able to help him partially. At this rate he believed all of his savings would be exhausted in another one and half years. One of the partners of his first company had opened a new company and was ready to employ him. Nagaraj was advised to take treatment and to join for work after he was cured. Nagaraj wanted to be cured and not to miss this opportunity of the job. He shed tears while describing this.

Nagaraj was about 5ft tall and 50 kgs weight. He was a soft-spoken person. He tried to make his neck straight and failed. He couldn't stop head nodding also. My examination didn't reveal any presence of physical problems. He had these problems for one and half years and even if it was psychological it could have caused permanent fibrosis in the neck muscles because of lack of action in those muscles. If that fibrosis had developed the fibrous part of the muscle had to be cut surgically. This was my first approach if there was fibrosis. I probed further to ascertain this. I found out that he didn't have this problem when he was asleep and also for some time in the mornings. He had no head nodding and torticollis in sleep and for some time in the mornings. Based on this information I concluded that there was no fibrosis and it was only psychological. It was clear that torticollis was psychological, but the doubt remained regarding his head nodding. In a neurological condition called Chorea such head nodding is present. I sent him for a neurological opinion and the neurologist ruled out any neurological problem including Chorea.

It was clear that Nagaraj's problems were psychological. Each part of the body is under the influence of the mind. When the disturbance in the mind increases it results in psychological illness. The mind can affect the body through the nervous system in two ways. The mind can affect through the cortical system of the brain and cause disturbance of voluntary muscles like in the case of Nagaraj. It can affect through mid-brain and affect involuntary nervous system and cause disturbance in functioning of cardiovascular, alimentary systems, etc. In Nagaraj's case the voluntary muscular system was affected. We call this as Hysteria. The next agenda was how to cure his problem.

Nagaraj had come here from another state for the sake of treatment. He had to get back and take up a new job that had been offered to him. I developed a road map of treatment for him. I decided three pronged treatment, viz:- Pharmacotherapy, Deconditioning therapy and psychotherapy. I prescribed anxiety reducing medicine (tranquilizer). Its action was temporary. The root cause of the problem was dealt in psychotherapy. He was subjected to Sedac (Sedative Current) treatment. In Hysteria the illness has secondary gain and it serves some purpose. This hidden or unconscious purpose was dealt in psychotherapy. In Sedac treatment a painful electric stimulus was given to both temple regions while the patient thought of his problem. The mind would associate this painful stimulus with the problem and would make it undesirable. This was given once daily for six days.

The root cause of the problem had to be treated in psychotherapy. Nagaraj was instructed to express whatever came to his mind without any inhibitions (free association as described elsewhere). The first task was to deal with his pessimism about the outcome of his illness. He had lost hopes. One should never loose hopes. When a person loses hopes the outcome will be bad. If he had lost hopes completely, he would have not come for treatment. I had to make this hope stronger by building up his confidence in the treatment. My commitment to his problem was a big hope to him. The confidence in the therapist automatically instills confidence in the patient. He had become pessimistic when he was not cured by many specialists. I understood his apathy and told him he had not been treated by a psychiatrist. This rekindled his hope.

He felt bad even though he worked honestly and never did anything wrong to anybody why he had problems in the jobs and illness. I asked him why he was connecting the two. He was a god-fearing person and believed if he did anything wrong god would punish. I told him that he had a problem and it was nothing to do with anything bad he did or didn't do. This is called as therapeutic split. He felt he shouldn't have been born at all. What was the point in repenting about the past? He was born already and should think of present and future only. He had a belief that his brothers might come for help if he was not cured on the one hand and he had a fear if they didn't come for help then what to do? We can sense the conflict here. He was already offered a job and why he should depend upon anybody else? He agreed and he should worry about his illness and its outcome.

Nagaraj expressed that he was not able to provide well to his family. He had a a bit of self-accusation for everything. He had done his best in what he could do, and he should feel happy about it. He was losing his self- confidence with any setbacks in life. Failures must be steppingstones for success. When there is failure one should try with more vigor and sooner or later, he will succeed. These had a positive effect on Nagaraj. Life is a struggle and people expect easy sailing. Nagaraj decided to fight against his problems and not to depend on anybody. There was a gradual improvement in him. His head nodding had stopped, and he was able to move his neck in all directions. I permitted him to take up his new job and report for a follow up after a month. He was happy and confident when he came for follow up. For two years he continued to see me whenever he visited his relatives here.

Psychodynamics

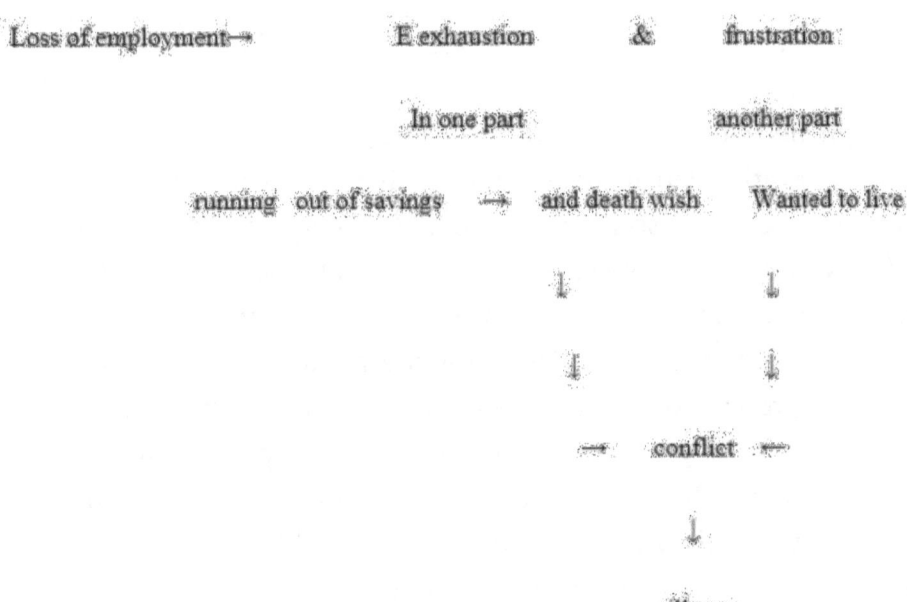

Let us look at the psychodynamics of Nagaraj's problem. A good and honest worker lost his job of twenty years for no fault of his.

In another job he was relieved to accommodate someone else. He was jobless for one and half years and exhausted about half of his savings. He had a responsibility to provide for the family. This stress was overwhelming for him. He lost his confidence and hope. At that time, he developed the above problems of back pain, head nodding and torticollis for one year. These developed after six months of unemployment. His frustrations led to death wishes. He was a good worker and was responsible for the family. He loved his family. We can sense the conflict here. On the one hand he was frustrated with death wishes and on the other hand he had a survival instinct to live and live for the family. The result of this conflict was his illness. The survival instinct didn't allow him to die but caused illness. The ultimate end of illness was death. That was exactly his unconscious mind was trying to accomplish.

Psychotherapy

The foremost thing in psychotherapy was to build his hope and confidence. He was made aware of his frustration about job. Even though he was a good worker he lost jobs for none of his faults. The frustration led to death wish. It is not unusual to have death wishes when a person is frustrated. He wanted to live, for his own life instinct and for the sake of family. This led to a conflict between death and life instincts. Being aware of his conflicts and unconscious actions resulted in cure. Nagaraj asked me an interesting question. Why his problem didn't disappear when he was offered a new job? In one year, his body and mind had become conditioned to the problem. Human being when once conditioned for something he doesn't want to give up. This was made to be undesirable by deconditioning therapy. The outcome was good. Still do you want to believe in age old adage of there is no cure for mental illness in this twenty first century.

Transgender

Roma a 26 years old lady was brought by her parents. For one month she had poor sleep, not eating well, just sitting and staring and engrossed in thoughts. About one and half years back she quit working because some boys were teasing her.

Roma a single person told me that she had no troubles, but she was ready to see me for treatment. This was a peculiar situation. Why a person with no problems would agree to see me for treatment. As a psychiatrist I would say there was a problem and she was not ready to reveal at that time. The very fact that she had no objection to see me indicated partial insight. At such times we should not be in a hurry to probe into the problem. Patience is required. I just ascertained that she had no physical problem. She was of more than average intelligence. Her higher mental functions were normal. She looked to be a shy and inhibited person. She was restless and depressed. I prescribed her an antidepressant and an antianxiety medicines and suggested her to see me after a week.

In the next two visits there was no progress in the treatment. She was not talking spontaneously. She would answer for any question in a single word saying "no". I could notice that she was very shy and inhibited. In the following visit she said that some boys stared at her. She denied that it was like harassing a girl. They never came even nearer her. Usually the attraction and appreciation of looks from opposite sex is adored by a person (at least internally, if not openly) and it is an instinct. She didn't think it was the case here. On the other hand, girls hate harassment from antisocial boys. She didn't think it was that also. The whole session was spent on trying to find out her feelings about boys staring at her. There was no answer by the end of the session.

In the next session she said those boys followed her. I tried to find out what it meant to her being followed by the boys. Boys following a girl are a very common happening. What she was trying to communicate was the question? Here we must find out whether she liked it or hated it. She again denied both. The whole session was spent on that and again ended up with no answer.

In the next session she said that those boys clapped their hands at her. She could not say what it meant to her. So far, she had talked about boys staring, following her and clapping at her. I told her that there must be some strong feelings that she had about it. She agreed, but what was that feeling remained a question. I tried to find out if it was a pleasant or unpleasant feeling. She said it was an unpleasant feeling. I asked her whether it was an embarrassing feeling. She confirmed it. One of the common comment's girls don't like is negative comments on their looks. She denied that (In fact she was good looking). Then I asked her what else about her looks that she thought could be embarrassing? After probing a lot, she said that those boys might be thinking that she was a transgender. Her response was very unusual one. Staring, following and clapping did it mean a transgender? For my question she said transgender meant that person was neither a boy nor a girl. She denied of ever feeling like that any time about herself. How did she know that was what they were feeling about her? At this stage I knew that she had some feelings about her looks, and she was not able to express. I asked her directly the feelings about her looks. She said that she loved her looks except for her height and weight. She mentioned that she was 5feet nine inches height and weighed 170 pounds. On my questioning she felt her weight and height were closer to a man's height and weight, but she didn't feel it was masculine. She felt it was odd for a girl. We can see the flow of thought pointing towards transgender. She felt her weight and height were not feminine and yet didn't feel masculine also. The result was transgender. She shyly confirmed that and almost cried.

Our society has laid down some unexpressed criteria for what is feminine and masculine. A woman with more height and weight is considered as somewhat like a man. There are so many women with even more height and weight of Roma. Why they don't feel like her was a question. She was able to accept that transgender was her own feeling about her looks. Biologically she was a woman. She was unhappy about her looks. I told her to accept that she was a woman and looks like height and weight cannot change her biological body constitution.

The boys stared, followed and clapped at her was true, but she misconstrued that they were teasing her as if she was a transgender. She accepted it was her assumption. She had subscribed to certain feelings of the society about femininity and masculinity. She accepted that she was biologically a woman with more than average height and weight. Her feelings about being a transgender vanished.

Psychodynamics

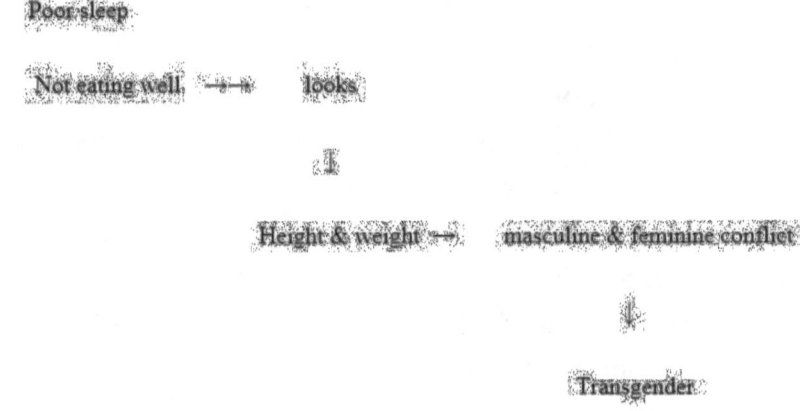

Roma came for poor sleep, not eating well and engrossed in her own thoughts. Roma had unhappy feelings about her height and weight. She felt she was not feminine because of her height and weights were closer to that of a man. On the one had she knew that she was a woman, but height and weight made her to feel that she was like a man. That concept of being a man was not acceptable to her mind again. A conflict generated and this turmoil led to her symptoms. Her mind unconsciously took a via media that is transgender. In society a woman is feminine if she is of less weight and height. If she is not feminine the only alternative is masculine, but she knew that she was not masculine. Then her mind created an entity in between man and a woman, i.e. transgender.

The boys were teasing her as usual like any other girl, but she construed it as if she was teasing her that she was a transgender. No one ever told her that she was a transgender explicitly. It was purely her own feeling. Unconsciously she herself had felt like a transgender. Girls usually enjoy positive comments on their beauty quietly. Why she misconstrued it as transgender? It is because she had unhappy opinion about her own weight and height.

Psychotherapy

It was very difficult to elicit from her any feelings. A lot had to be probed and repeated questioning led to her disclosure of feelings. We must understand that it was not easy for her to disclose such a painful feeling. Her wrong opinion about weight and height for men and women had to be made aware to her. She accepted it was a wrong opinion on her part. She was made aware that she was biologically a woman and just thinking otherwise won't change the truth. A woman should not judge femininity or masculinity based on height and weight. This we call as therapeutic split. She began accepting that she was a woman, no matter what her weight and height were.

Psychotherapy took place in sixteen sessions. It took longer than usual, because she was less communicative, and feelings had to be extracted from her with repeated questioning. Psychotherapy is usually faster in a well communicating individual.

Bipolar Disorder

Gaurav, a 35 years old married male with two children was referred to me by a doctor. Gaurav was ill for about 5 years. He had treatment from two psychiatrists already. The problem was continuing. He was accompanied by his wife and both of his parents. They had brought big file about his treatment. They told me that Gaurav was repeatedly getting sick. They said that he had high and low attacks (These were their words). Later I came to know that at times he would become highly energetic (High attacks) and did a lot of things in a short period of time. Some other times he would seclude and avoided everybody and stayed alone in the room (low attacks).

I interviewed Gaurav. Gaurav Was a Bachelor of Engineering graduate and worked in a state government organization as a civil engineer. He was a topper in engineering college. He did not report any family problems. He married his wife about seven years ago. It was an arranged marriage, and both got along very well. He had one son of one-year age. The son, his wife and both parents were healthy. Theirs was a happy family. His father had a boutique and was earning well. Gaurav had good salary. Theirs was a joint family and all got along well with each other.

After knowing all the above everyone would wonder why Gaurav was ill. I talked to Gaurav alone. He was eloquent and talkative. He said that he did not know why he was falling ill so many times. He could not identify any reason for it. He was very unhappy about it. He had five high attacks and three low attacks in five years. He had those attacks gradually. When he had high attacks, he was very energetic and could accomplish so many things in a short time. At those times he was a hero for everybody. He would venture into too many things and finally ended up leaving them in the middle. This resulted in heavy loss to the family. At that stage everybody cursed and advised him. When he had low attacks, he became depressed, was not going to work properly, remained in his room, not meeting anyone, not eating and not sleeping properly. His both attacks lasted anywhere from two months to five months. In between the attacks he was completely alright. His higher mental functions were alright.

I made a diagnosis of Manic-depressive disorder. I reviewed his treatment files and the previous psychiatrists had made the same diagnosis. The medicines given were correct. I had to ascertain why he was not cured despite good treatments so far. The most common thing in our society is poor follow up. This was the case in Gaurav also. He was taking medicines till he was better and stopped them without even consulting the doctor. I found out even the earlier doctors had told him the importance of proper follow up. He and the family felt that he was better, and doctors were just trying to make money by unnecessarily continuing the treatment. They had discontinued the treatment on their own.

I told him and the family that earlier doctors were right, and they had given good treatment. They should go back to their doctor and follow up the treatment. They didn't want to face their doctors out of guilt. They preferred to be treated by me. I informed them not to repeat improper follow up this time. If one allowed the illness to flare up repeatedly it might become chronic and It required a very long time treatment, perhaps for years. His illness was well under control with medicines and they should not spoil it. All these had an impact on them.

He was under my treatment for about nine years and he did not have even a single attack. He was transferred elsewhere, and he promised to continue treatment in a new place. Manic depressive disorder is quite a common disease. It affects usually young adults. In a typical case there are manic (high) and depressive (low) attacks. In some there may be only manic or depressive attacks. After the manic or depressive attacks are treated, they require mood stabilizers. This disorder is mainly because of biochemical changes in the body. There may be some genetic factor (recessive gene) in some. The treatment here is mainly pharmacotherapy.

Do You Have A Mental Illness?

Everybody gets this question many times in their lives. Nobody expresses it to others, because of the fear of being labeled as mad. I have observed people discuss frankly about mind and mental illness. They say mind is very important. They say that mind is powerful and admit it has an impact on the body. People think that mental illness is synonymous with madness. In mental illnesses there are minor, medium and major illnesses just like it is in physical illnesses. In my practice 90% of patients that I see are minor and medium illnesses like neurosis, depression, etc. Only about 10% are major illnesses like Schizophrenia, Manic depressive illness, etc. A lot of them know that a vast majority people's physical problem are deep rooted in mind. Yet they hesitate to seek a psychiatric consultation because of stigma and ignorance. The very same people if one complains his mind is not under control they label him as "his screw is loose". It means madness. This is the kind of social stigma prevailing n the society.

Human being has both mind and body. In any illness one should keep both mind and body as to the causative relationship. There are purely physical and mental illnesses also. More than 50% of all physical symptoms are caused by the problems in the mind. Some patient think that they have a physical illness and when it is not cured with best treatment they are puzzled about the illness. Some may even take refuge to fate. In such cases there may be underlying psychological problems. The outcome of the treatment will be better if coupled with psychiatric care also. Because of the fear of being labeled as madness people are afraid to seek psychiatric help. Of course, they can seek help confidentially, but they hesitate because of their own stigma about mental illness. When they visit a psychiatrist, they are always afraid if somebody notices them. If some other person sees them, they are afraid their family reputation will go. If the word spreads that someone has seen a psychiatrist one will have difficulty in finding a matrimonial alliance, etc. If one sees a psychiatrist, it doesn't mean he is mad. I have been in psychiatric practice for more than 4 decades. I have seen a lot of changes in people's attitude towards mental illness in 4 decades. Our society is accepting it better than before, yet social stigma is rampant. The question arises as to when to consider psychological problems need intervention. Here I have written some symptoms and signs below, which may help you to decide if one needs any treatment. It may not clear all the doubts in readers minds, if in doubt don't hesitate to get an opinion from a psychiatrist.

1. sleep problems
2. anxiety and fear
3. worries & depression
4. shyness
5. impatience
6. suspicion and jealousness
7. poor appetite
8. headache
9. frequently changing jobs
10. underachievement
11. disturbing dreams

12. unable to say no to people
13. alcohol, drug abuse and social media habituation
14. Sexual problems
15. Indecisiveness
16. Over protectiveness of children
17. Irritable over small matters
18. Unable to express emotions
19. Inability to enjoy some free time
20. Not able to make friends
21. Not mingling with anybody and loneliness
22. Frequent injuries
23. Sudden change in behavior
24. Suicide and deathwishes
25. Repeated thoughts and actions (obsessions and compulsions)
26. Unable to accept aging and behaving like a younger person
27. Excessive cursing themselves or others
28. Hearing voices or having visions (hallucinations)
29. False beliefs (delusions)
30. Fear of disease or death
31. Fear the whole world is bad and everyone is a cheat
32. Excessive tiredness
33. Hysterical paralysis
34. Even when a doctor says there is no illness and still believing he has illness (hypochondriasis)

35. When a real physical illness has not responded to a best treatment

36. Sleep walking (somnambulism)

37. Some physical illnesses are deeply rooted in psychological factors like duodenal ulcer, blood pressure, etc.

All the above are symptoms and signs of psychological illness. The presence of these symptoms and signs do not mean one has psychological illness. WHO has laid down certain guidelines for a mental illness? The above signs and symptoms should be to the extent of causing severe disability in functioning in any area of life like familial, educational, vocational, social, physical spheres. All people have one or more of the above symptoms. It may not be mental illness and it may not need treatment. Causing severe disturbance in area of functioning in life is the criteria.

When once one decides to seek treatment, the question arises as to whom one should see. Often people do not know the difference between a psychiatrist, neurologist and neurosurgeon. A psychiatrist deals with only psychological problems. A neurologist provides care for neurological diseases. There is definite pathology in nervous system in neurological diseases. A neurosurgeon carries out surgery on the pathological nervous system.

Often people are confused about the difference between psychiatrist, psychologist, social worker and psychiatric nurse. A psychiatrist has a basic degree in medicine (MBBS) and then specializes in psychiatry. A psychologist has a degree (BA, MS, Phd) in psychology. A social worker has a degree (MSW) in social work. Psychiatric nurse takes care of the patient under the supervision of the psychiatrist. A psychiatrist treats the patients. A psychologist carries out the necessary psychological testing. A social worker collects necessary information relating to the problem of the patient.

There are clinical psychologists involved in testing as well as treating patients.

There are different approaches in the treatment of mentally ill as below: -

a) Psychotherapy: - It is also known as talk therapy and counseling amongst general public. There are different types in psychotherapy. In psychodynamic psychotherapy, the mind dynamics are explored, and relief given. When once the patient is aware of his problem, he will be able to cope with them by altering his behavior. There is supportive psychotherapy, marital psychotherapy etc.

b) Behavioral therapy: - a certain behavior can be modified by reward and punishment, etc.

c) Psycho pharmacotherapy: - The various medicines are used in the treatment. There is a tremendous advance in this nowadays.

d) Physical therapy: - Electro convulsive therapy was in use a lot in earlier days. Now its use is restricted to only to a few resistant cases.

e) Cognitive therapy: - helps in developing skills and modifying beliefs.

These are some commonly used therapies. As science advances newer therapies will emerge.

The mind undergoes development from birth. There are studies to demonstrate mind begins to develop even in mother's womb. It has been observed that the fetus will have vigorous movements if the mother is in the site of a fight. On the other hand, if mother is listening to a soft music the fetus has fewer movements.

Initially the child is full of instincts. This stage is known as ID. The parents are the most important for the earlier development of the mind. Grand parents, teachers and others also play a role. Child's interaction with them lays the foundation for the personality development. The values of the society is inculcated by the child and this results in development of superego. The interaction between ID (Instincts) and Superego leads to the development of Ego. In a healthy individual a strong development of Ego is important in order to lead a harmonious life. The innate constitution of the individual also plays a part in the development. The life's good incidences will have a bearing on the development of the mind. On other hand unhappy incidences may be buried in the unconscious mind. This may result in a conflict and cause problems.

Mind is very powerful. It has effect on every part of the body, if ignored it may lead to a lot of problems. The adage, which says that "there is no medicine for mental illness" is no longer true and it is a myth.

About the Author

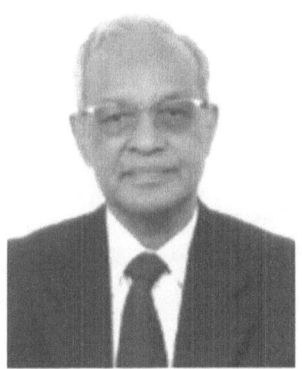

Dr K M Druva Kumar is a retired psychiatrist in Bangalore with 45 years' experience. He has written this book for the general public. The purpose of the book was to thwart stigma and ignorance on mental illness. He has selected the most commonly occurring psychiatric problems. He has narrated actual case examples while taking care of confidentiality of the patient.

He graduated from medical college, Mysore. Then he was a resident, fellow and a faculty at Detroit Psychiatric Institute (DPI) of Wayne state university school of medicine, Detroit, Michigan. He was a director of one division of DPI. He was the first Indian to be admitted to Michigan psychoanalytic institute, Detroit. He became a board-certified psychiatrist in 1976.

He returned to India in 1976 and practiced in Bangalore. He was a president of Indian psychiatric society-Karnataka branch (IPS-KB). He was declared as Eminent Psychiatrist by IPS-KB in 1982. He was the chairman for annual conference of IPS-KB in 1982. He was recipient of Community leaders of America award in 1972. He was the recipient of Dr LGP Achar, Dr S S Jayaram, Eminent psychiatrist and senior psychiatrist awards of IPS-KB. He also has two rotary awards. He is a fellow member of Indian psychiatric society. He is corresponding member of American psychiatric association.

He had written articles on mental illness in kannada Kasturi digest. He compiled them and brought out a book "Manoviplava".

www.ingramcontent.com/pod-product-compliance
Lightning Source LLC
Chambersburg PA
CBHW030924180526
45163CB00002B/452